MW00950802

THE NEW
AUTOIMMUNE
Protocol Diet
COOKBOOK FOR BEGINNERS

Anti-Inflammatory, Healing and Tasty Recipes to Balance
Your Immune System and Boost Gut Health |
Includes Expert Advice & a 28-Day Meal Plan

Amelia Patel

Copyright © 2024 by Amelia Patel.

All rights reserved. No part of this publication may be reproduced, distributed or transmitted in any form or by any means, electronic or mechanical, including photocopying, recording or by any information storage and retrieval system, without permission in writing from the author, except in the case of brief quotations embodied in critical reviews and certain other noncommercial uses permitted by copyright law.

Legal Notice:

This is a legal notice to inform you that the book titled THE NEW AUTOIMMUNE PROTOCOL DIET COOKBOOK FOR BEGINNERS authored by Amelia Patel is protected by copyright law. Any unauthorized distribution, reproduction, or use the book, in whole or in part, is strictly prohibited and may result in legal action being taken against you. Under the copyright law, the author has the exclusive right to reproduce, distribute, and publicly display the book. Any use of the book without the permission of the author or the publisher is a violation of their legal rights.

Disclaimer Notice:

The book titled THE NEW AUTOIMMUNE PROTOCOL DIET COOKBOOK FOR BEGINNERS by Amelia Patel is provided for informational purposes only. The recipes contained in this book are the result of the author's own experiences and preferences and any may not be suitable for all readers. The author has taken every effort to ensure that the recipes contained in this book are accurate and up to date at the time of publication. However, the author and publisher make no warranties or representations, express or implied, as to the accuracy or completeness of the information contained herein. The author and publisher will not be liable for any damages or injuries arising from the use of the information contained in this book or from any errors or omissions in the content of the book. The reader assumes all responsibility for the use of the information contained in this book. The author and publisher reserve the right to make changes to the content of this book at any time without notice.

Readers are advised to consult a qualified healthcare professional for diagnosis and treatment of any medical condition and before starting any new health regimen. The author and publisher have made every effort to ensure the accuracy and completeness of the information presented herein, but they assume no responsibility for errors, omission or interpretations of the subject matter.

By reading this book, you agree to the terms of this disclaimer notice. If you do not agree with these terms, you should not read or use this book.

TABLE OF CONTENTS

FOREWORD

‎———

I t gives me great pleasure to present to you *The New Autoimmune Protocol Diet Cookbook*. As an integrative nutritionist and expert in autoimmune disease management through nutrition, I have seen firsthand how profoundly the Autoimmune Protocol diet can help those suffering from chronic inflammation and autoimmunity. However, following such a specialized diet plan can be challenging without the right guidance and recipe resources. That is why I set out to create this comprehensive cookbook - to provide anyone following the AIP diet with over 100 recipes, meal plans, and substitution guides to make their healing journey smooth and delicious.

The Autoimmune Protocol, commonly known as AIP, is an elimination diet designed to reduce overall inflammation levels and heal gut function. By removing common trigger foods that can disrupt gut barrier function and the immune system, the AIP diet allows the body to regain balance and calm a hyperactive immune response. Although elimination diets can feel restrictive at first, my goal with this cookbook was to showcase how AIP-compliant eating can still be nutritious, satisfying, and full of flavors from around the world. You will find recipes featuring grass-fed beef, wild-caught fish, antioxidant-rich vegetables, immune-supportive herbs and spices, nourishing fats, and more—all aligned with the strictest AIP guidelines.

In the introductory chapters, I have provided an in-depth look at how the immune system functions, what goes awry to cause autoimmunity, and the impact of chronic inflammation and leaky gut on long-term health. You will learn how addressing underlying gut dysbiosis and restoring gut barrier integrity is crucial for attenuating autoimmune disease activity naturally over time. I will explain the phases of the AIP diet and how it supports overall immune regulation and gut healing through the targeted elimination of common food allergens. You will also gain a solid understanding of the key supplements and lifestyle factors that can enhance healing when following an AIP-centric approach.

The recipes themselves have been carefully developed to support the various stages of the AIP reintroduction process. Throughout the cookbook, you will find recipes for breakfast favorites like coconut yogurt parfaits and grain-free waffles, hearty salads and vegetarian main dishes, anti-inflammatory fish and meat preparations, satisfying snacks, and even nourishing desserts. All recipes call for whole, unprocessed ingredients and emphasize immune-modulating spices, herbs, healthy fats, and polyphenol-rich vegetables and fruits. You'll also find chapters dedicated to gut-supportive bone broths, fermented foods, and various healing condiments and sauces. A comprehensive 28-day meal plan is provided to help you confidently navigate your first month of AIP.

In the appendices, you will find invaluable resources, including an exhaustive grocery shopping checklist, food swap guides, and measurement conversion charts. My goal was to address any question or challenge you may face when adopting this healing lifestyle long-term. I hope The Autoimmune Protocol Diet Cookbook serves as your nourishing and comprehensive daily companion throughout your autoimmune health journey. By following these science-backed dietary principles alongside this recipe guidance, I am confident you will experience lasting relief from chronic symptoms naturally over time. But most of all, I hope you find the AIP way of eating to be sustainable, satisfying and enjoyable for years to come. Bon appétit!

Chapter 1

INTRODUCTION TO THE AUTOIMMUNE DIET

In this first chapter, we will explore the basic workings of the immune system and what happens to cause its dysfunction in autoimmune disease. Our immune system has evolved to protect us from pathogens and foreign invaders in the environment through the coordinated efforts of both the innate and adaptive immune responses. White blood cells, cytokines, antibodies and more all work together harmoniously via cells like T cells, B cells and macrophages to fend off infection on a daily basis. However, in the case of autoimmunity, the immune system fails to properly distinguish self from non-self and mistakenly attacks healthy tissues in the body. The root causes behind this loss of tolerance are multifactorial but revolve around a dysfunctional immune response coupled with a disturbed gut microbiome and permeable intestinal wall, leading to chronic systemic inflammation.

Understanding normal immune physiology provides necessary context to appreciate what veers off course to result in autoimmune pathological states. We will explore the leading hypotheses around what sparks or sustains autoimmune disturbances, such as potential roles for genetics, gut dysbiosis, environmental triggers and the emerging microbiome-gut-brain axis. By the end of this chapter, you will gain insights into why autoimmune diseases are so complex and challenging to treat using conventional methods alone, laying the groundwork for later discussions around targeted dietary interventions like the Autoimmune Protocol.

1.1. HOW THE IMMUNE SYSTEM WORKS

The human immune system is a complex network of specialized cells, tissues, and organs that work together to defend against infecting microorganisms and other foreign invaders. It is arguably one of the most intricate and finely tuned physiological systems within the human body. In this extensive overview, we will examine the multiple layers that comprise the immune system and how they function in ˙seamless coordination to protect our health on a daily basis.

The First Line of Defense: Innate Immunity

Innate immunity, also known as non-specific immunity, encompasses the body's immediate defenses that react to pathogens in a generic manner. The main players of the innate immune system include physical and chemical barriers, phagocytic cells, and signaling molecules known as cytokines.

Physical and Chemical Barriers

Physical barriers like skin and mucous membranes provide a mechanical blockade against invading microbes. The skin acts as an impermeable layer shielding the body from harmful external pathogens and substances. Mucous membranes lining various hollow organs secrete mucus, which traps and sweeps away potential pathogens. Additionally, tears produced by the eyes and mucus in the nose and airways help wash away foreign particles.

Chemical barriers include substances like stomach acid which creates an acidic environment toxic to most organisms. The stomach produces hydrochloric acid maintaining a pH level between 1-2, which kills the majority of microbes that enter through the digestive tract. Other secretions such as lysozyme in tears and saliva contain enzymes that can break down cell walls of certain bacteria. Together, these physical and chemical barriers comprise a formidable first line of defense.

Phagocytic Cells

Should a pathogen breach these initial barriers, phagocytic cells spring into action. Neutrophils are key players and are usually the first white blood cells to arrive at infection sites within hours. They engulf microbes through phagocytosis, a complex process involving cell membrane extension, engulfment and formation of a phagosome which then fuses with lysosomes. Microbial degradation and disposal is achieved through the release of antimicrobial enzymes from phagolysosomes.

Macrophages are resident tissue phagocytes that participate in both immune activation and regulation. They recognize broad classes of pathogens through pattern recognition receptors and induce inflammatory responses. As professional antigen presenting cells, macrophages can also process engulfed pathogens and present pieces on MHC molecules to activate lymphocytes of the adaptive immune system.

Adaptive Immunity: Targeted Defenses

Should innate immune defenses prove inadequate to clear an invading pathogen, a highly specialized second line of targeted defense arises through adaptive immunity. Also known as acquired immunity, this arm creates immunological memory through antigen exposure to mount an accelerated response upon future encounters.

Humoral Immunity

B cells play a major role in humoral immunity through antibody production. Antibodies, also known as immunoglobulins, are Y-shaped glycoproteins released by plasma blasts and plasma cells in response to foreign pathogens. There are five major classes of antibodies (IgG, IgM, IgA, IgE, IgD) which play distinct yet complementary roles in neutralizing microbes. IgG is the most abundant antibody in the blood and extracellular fluid which can activate compliment pathways. IgM is the first antibody produced during initial infections.

Upon recognition of antigen with their B cell receptors, B cells become activated and begin proliferating rapidly. They receive signals from helper T cells to mature and differentiate into either memory B cells for long-term protection, or antibody secreting plasma cells. Antibodies tag pathogens for destruction via various methods and provide the basis for hallmark diagnostic tests.

Cell-Mediated Immunity

T cells direct cell-mediated responses against infections. Two major types of T cells enact this immunity. Cytotoxic "killer" T cells seek and destroy virally-infected cells or tumor cells with help from helper T cells. Recognition occurs through binding of the T cell receptor to virally-derived peptide fragments presented on MHC class I molecules.

Helper T cells activate and regulate both arms of adaptive immunity. They express CD4 co-receptors enabling recognition of foreign peptides in the context of MHC class II on antigen presenting cells. Upon activation, helpers secrete cytokines stimulating B cell antibody production, activation of cytotoxic T cells, recruitment of phagocytes and expression of cell surface molecules by various immune cells.

Antigens: The Fingerprints of Pathogens

All adaptive immune responses precisely recognize foreign substances called antigens that are presented on major histocompatibility complex (MHC) molecules. Antigens constitute the molecular "fingerprints" unique to each pathogen and can take the form of macromolecules like proteins/peptides, polysaccharides or lipids. There are two main pathways for antigen presentation:

Extracellular Antigen Presentation

The extracellular or exogenous route involves professional antigen presenting cells (APCs) like macrophages and dendritic cells internalizing pathogens via phagocytosis or endocytosis. Within these cells, the pathogens are broken down through proteolysis into smaller protein fragments. Select fragments bind to MHC class II molecules and are transported to the cell surface for recognition by CD4+ T helper cells.

This pathway aids clearance of extracellular bacteria and parasites. It also drives production of pathogen-specific antibodies by activating B cells when they receive costimulatory signals from CD4+ T cells.

Intracellular Antigen Presentation

The intracellular or endogenous route occurs when viruses or some bacteria infect cells and begin replicating within the cytosol. As new virus particles are assembled, they produce viral antigens. These antigens are then fed into the cytosolic degradation pathways where they are broken into peptides.

The antigenic peptides bind to MHC class I molecules and are expressed on the infected cell surface. There, they can be recognized by CD8+ cytotoxic T lymphocytes whose role is to identify and eliminate infected cells. This helps control viruses that evade extracellular defenses and hijack host cells to replicate.

Together, these dual antigen presentation pathways allow the adaptive immune system to mount tailored responses based on the unique molecular signatures of diverse pathogens. Precision recognition of antigens initiates highly-targeted defenses minimizing collateral damage to host tissues.

Mounting an Adaptive Attack

Clonal Expansion and Differentiation

Upon recognition of cognate antigen, naive T and B cells proliferate extensively through cell division. This clonal expansion leads to thousands or millions of daughter cells specific for the pathogen. Effector T cells develop based on localized cytokine signals, taking forms like TH1, TH2, or cytotoxic CD8+ cells tailored to the invading microbe. Activated B cells differentiate into short-lived plasma cells or memory B cells.

Effector Functions

Plasma cells rapidly secrete high levels of pathogen-specific antibodies into circulation or tissues. These Y-shaped proteins can neutralize toxins or coat pathogens for ingestion by phagocytes. Activated macrophages and cytotoxic T cells enhance microbial killing through release of toxic radicals and granules. Cytokines coordinate the appropriate response, with IFN-γ enhancing macrophage microbicidal activity against viruses and intracellular bacteria.

Memory Formation

A fraction of effector T and B cell clones evade apoptosis and transition into long-lived memory cell populations. Memory T cells patrol through circulation or tissues for years. Upon re-exposure, they rapidly perform recall responses preventing symptomatic infection through robust clonal expansion and more potent effector functions than during primary exposure. This immunological memory provides the basis for successful vaccination strategies.

Through Innate Priming, Clonal Selection, Effector Mechanisms and Memory Formation, the immune system has evolved a sophisticated adaptive response tailored against pathogens over a lifetime of repeated exposures and challenges. Continued study of these mechanisms informs new therapeutic approaches against diseases.

1.2. UNDERSTANDING AUTOIMMUNE DISEASES

In any healthy immune system, a delicate balance is maintained between reacting robustly to pathogens while simultaneously avoiding responses against the body's own healthy cells and tissues. Autoimmune diseases occur when this tolerance breaks down, causing the immune system to mistakenly attack and damage self-components. In this extensive overview, we will explore the underlying mechanisms behind various autoimmune conditions and gain greater insights into these debilitating illnesses.

The Spectrum of Autoimmunity

Varied Presentations

Autoimmune diseases can affect nearly every organ system and present with a wide range of symptoms, from mild fatigue to life-threatening organ failure. Clinical manifestations depend on the targeted antigens and tissues involved. While each disease has distinguishing features, many share immunological characteristics.

Genetic and Environmental Influences

Both inherited genes and external exposures shape individual autoimmunity risk. Certain HLA alleles confer higher risk for particular diseases. Environmental triggers like infectious agents, toxins or medications may ignite pathogenic immune responses in genetically susceptible individuals.

Disruptions to Tolerance

Regardless of cause, the pathogenic mechanism underlying all autoimmunity involves a loss of self-tolerance, where self-reactive lymphocytes escape deletion or regulation in the thymus or periphery. This allows autoreactive cells and antibodies to attack self-antigens.

Gender and Hormonal Effects

Many autoimmune diseases preferentially affect women and symptoms often fluctuate with hormonal changes. Sex hormones like estrogen are thought to influence immune cell function and tolerance mechanisms beginning in early development.

Microbial Influences

The microbiota supports immune education and induction of tolerogenic responses. Microbial dysbiosis may enable expansion of self-reactive clones predisposed by genetic or toxic insults. Probiotics show promise restoring eubiosis.

Understanding the nuanced interplay between genetic predisposition and environmental influences sheds light on disease development and informs prevention and treatment strategies tailored to individual biomarkers and triggers.

Breakdown of Self-Tolerance

Self-tolerance is a critical mechanism that prevents the immune system from attacking the body's own tissues. In autoimmune diseases, this tolerance breaks down, leading to harmful immune responses against self-antigens. Recent research has identified several key factors contributing to this breakdown, including genetic predisposition, environmental triggers, and dysregulation of immune checkpoints. For instance, a 2023 study published in Nature Immunology highlighted the role of T cell exhaustion in the loss of self-tolerance, suggesting new therapeutic targets for autoimmune disorders.

Central Tolerance Mechanisms

Central tolerance occurs primarily in the thymus for T cells and the bone marrow for B cells. During this process, developing lymphocytes that strongly react to self-antigens are eliminated or reprogrammed. However, this system isn't perfect. Recent findings have shown that alterations in the autoimmune regulator (AIRE) gene can lead to defective central tolerance. A 2022 study in Immunity revealed that AIRE mutations not only affect T cell selection but also impact the development of regulatory T cells, crucial for maintaining peripheral tolerance.

Breaches in Peripheral Tolerance

Peripheral tolerance acts as a backup system to control autoreactive cells that escape central tolerance. It involves mechanisms like anergy, deletion, and suppression by regulatory T cells. However, these mechanisms can fail due to various factors. Recent research has focused on the role of checkpoint molecules like PD-1 and CTLA-4 in maintaining peripheral tolerance. A 2024 study in Science Translational Medicine demonstrated that targeted modulation of these checkpoints could potentially restore tolerance in autoimmune conditions.

Pathogenic Autoimmunity Emerges

When tolerance mechanisms fail, autoreactive lymphocytes can become activated and attack self-tissues. This process involves complex interactions between various immune cells and inflammatory mediators.

Recent advances in single-cell sequencing have provided unprecedented insights into the heterogeneity of autoreactive cells. A 2023 Nature study used this technology to identify specific T cell subsets responsible for tissue damage in rheumatoid arthritis, opening new avenues for targeted therapies.

Progression of Autoimmune Disease

Autoimmune diseases often follow a relapsing-remitting course or progress gradually over time. The mechanisms underlying these patterns are still being elucidated. Recent long-term studies have revealed that chronic inflammation can lead to epigenetic changes in both immune and tissue cells, perpetuating the disease. A 2024 review in Nature Reviews Immunology highlighted how these epigenetic alterations could explain the persistence of autoimmunity even after apparent remission.

Factors Contributing to Tolerance Defects

Multiple factors contribute to tolerance breakdown, including genetics, environment, and lifestyle. Recent genome-wide association studies have identified numerous risk loci for various autoimmune diseases. Additionally, the role of the microbiome in shaping immune tolerance has gained significant attention. A 2023 Cell study demonstrated how specific gut bacteria could influence regulatory T cell function, potentially explaining the link between diet and autoimmunity.

Restoring Self-Tolerance Remains a Goal

Efforts to restore self-tolerance represent a promising approach to treating autoimmune diseases. Recent clinical trials have explored various strategies, including antigen-specific therapies and cellular therapies using regulatory T cells. A 2024 New England Journal of Medicine study reported promising results from a phase II trial using engineered regulatory T cells to treat type 1 diabetes, showcasing the potential of tolerance-inducing therapies.

Target Organs in Autoimmunity

Autoimmune diseases can affect various organs and tissues throughout the body, with each condition targeting specific structures. Recent research has provided deeper insights into the mechanisms of organ-specific autoimmune damage:

Thyroid (Hashimoto's Thyroiditis)

In Hashimoto's thyroiditis, autoantibodies primarily target thyroid peroxidase (TPO) and thyroglobulin. A 2023 study in Nature Immunology revealed that these antibodies not only cause direct damage but also activate complement cascades, amplifying inflammation. The research also identified a subset of thyroid-infiltrating T cells that secrete interferon-gamma, contributing to ongoing tissue destruction.

Joints (Rheumatoid Arthritis)

Rheumatoid arthritis (RA) primarily affects synovial joints. Recent findings have expanded our understanding beyond rheumatoid factor. A 2024 Arthritis & Rheumatology study demonstrated that anti-citrullinated protein antibodies (ACPAs) play a crucial role in bone erosion by directly activating osteoclasts. Additionally, the study identified a novel fibroblast subtype in the synovium that drives persistent inflammation even after initial immune triggers subside.

Nervous System (Multiple Sclerosis)

Multiple sclerosis (MS) involves immune-mediated damage to the central nervous system's myelin sheaths. A groundbreaking 2023 Brain study used advanced imaging techniques to show that B cells, not just T cells, can directly contribute to myelin damage. The research also revealed that some autoantibodies in MS patients target specific potassium channels on neurons, explaining some of the non-myelin-related symptoms.

Pancreatic Islets (Type 1 Diabetes)

Type 1 diabetes results from the autoimmune destruction of insulin-producing beta cells. A 2024 Cell Metabolism study uncovered a previously unknown interaction between autoreactive T cells and pancreatic stellate cells, which exacerbates islet inflammation. The research also identified a subset of regulatory T cells that, when properly stimulated, can protect beta cells from autoimmune attack, offering new therapeutic possibilities.

Skin (Psoriasis)

Psoriasis is characterized by T cell-driven inflammation leading to keratinocyte hyperproliferation. A 2023 Journal of Investigative Dermatology study revealed that IL-23-producing dendritic cells in psoriatic lesions have a unique transcriptional profile, making them key drivers of pathogenic T cell responses. The study also demonstrated how these cells interact with the skin microbiome, potentially explaining why certain infections can trigger psoriasis flares.

These recent findings highlight the complexity of organ-specific autoimmune processes and offer new targets for therapeutic interventions. They underscore the importance of considering the unique microenvironment of each affected organ in developing targeted treatments for autoimmune diseases.

Immune System Dysregulation in Autoimmunity

Chronic activation of both innate and adaptive immunity sustains long-term self-attack. Dendritic cells present self-antigens with reduced regulatory signaling. Macrophages secrete excess inflammatory cytokines like TNF-α. Presentation of ubiquitously expressed self-antigens to naïve CD4+ T cells promotes their pathogenic polarization to pro-inflammatory Th1/Th17 subsets.

Helper T cells not only stimulate autoreactive B cells to secrete autoantibodies but also recruit monocytes, neutrophils and natural killer cells into affected tissues. Loss of regulatory T cell populations further disrupts immunological self-tolerance leaving pathology unchecked. Dysfunctional immune regulation and self-antigen presentation are pivotal drivers of autoimmunity across diverse clinical manifestations.

Promoting Remission Through a Personalized Lens

As our understanding of autoimmune mechanisms deepens, treatment approaches aim to restore tolerance, calm dysregulated immunity and limit end-organ damage through precision targeting. Therapies may variably involve immunosuppressants, biologics, targeted synthetic DMARDs, dietary/lifestyle changes or use of regenerative approaches depending on factors like disease stage and individual biomarker profiles. Adopting a personalized lens optimizes managing these heterogeneous lifelong conditions for improved quality of life.

1.3. CHRONIC INFLAMMATION AND AUTOIMMUNITY

Inflammation serves vital protective functions when initiated acutely by the immune system in response to pathogens, injuries or toxins. However, when this physiological reaction becomes persistently dysregulated and inappropriately targeted against the body's own tissues, a pathogenic state of chronic inflammation ensues with serious consequences. This section will explore the deep connections between chronic inflammation and the development of autoimmune diseases.

Acute vs Chronic Inflammation

Acute Inflammation

An acute response elicits redness, swelling, heat and pain via histamine, bradykinin and other inflammatory mediators released within hours. Improved blood flow recruits phagocytes to damaged sites. Fever and other symptoms isolate and disable invading pathogens. Resolution commences once triggers are eliminated via anti-inflammatory pathways.

Chronic Inflammation

Prolonged exposure to triggers prevents acute response resolution. Chronic cellular mediators like TNF-α, IL-1β and IL-6 predominate over regulatory cytokines long-term. Unresolved inflammation causes ongoing tissue damage as phagocytes release oxidants and enzymes. Chronic inflammation associates with age-related disease.

Underlying Causes

Obesity, infections, genetics and environmental toxins may chronically activate innate immune pattern recognition receptors. Subclinical microbial translocation, a dysbiotic microbiome or accumulated advanced glycation end products also sustain chronic inflammation.

Cellular Players

Macrophages, lymphocytes and fibroblasts create a localized self-perpetuating inflammatory milieu. Adaptive immunity aids resolution of acute inflammation but chronically activated T cells fail tolerance and resolution checkpoints.

Clinical Consequences

Protracted endothelial dysfunction and oxidative stress impact every organ system over decades. Chronic inflammation drives atherosclerosis, neurodegeneration, cancer and autoimmunity beyond initial triggers. Resolution pathways represent therapeutic targets.

Molecular Basis of Chronic Inflammation

NF-κB Pathway Dysregulation

The NF-κB transcription factor regulates hundreds of pro-inflammatory genes. Persistent activation leads to chronic overexpression of cytokines, enzymes and adhesion molecules within inflamed tissues. Failure to terminate NF-κB signaling sustains autoinflammation.

Elevated Inflammasome Activity

Inflammasomes like NLRP3 excessively process pro-inflammatory cytokines IL-1β and IL-18 when abnormally activated. Chronic inflammasome signaling amplifies inflammation through direct and indirect pathways.

Hyperresponsive Pattern Recognition

Toll-like receptors normally detect microbial ligands but respond similarly to damage signals. Sustained endogenous ligand binding maintains tissue inflammation as TLRs activate NF-κB and inflammasomes.

Transcriptomic Shock

Prolonged dysregulation of key pathways upregulates a pro-inflammatory gene expression profile. Anti-inflammatory compensatory mechanisms are overwhelmed.

Cellular Autocrine/Paracrine Effects

Immune cells secrete inflammatory mediators acting on themselves and other nearby cells in paracrine/autocrine feedback loops perpetuating the process.

Therapeutic strategies aim to interrupt these molecular drivers restoring balanced pro- and anti-inflammatory signaling resolution. Combination targeting may be required due to compensatory pathway activation.

Connection with Autoimmunity

Priming of the Immune System

Constant inflammatory mediators like TNF-α, IL-1β and IL-6 sensitize tissues, endothelium and antigen-presenting cells through prolonged receptor ligation. This upregulates adhesion molecules, co-stimulatory signals and alters transcription factor signaling priming cells for excessive activation. Sensitized tissues are more responsive to injury signals, further lowering activation thresholds for immune cells.

Loss of Regulatory Control

Excess glucocorticoids released under chronic stress fail to restrain inflammation once Feedback dissipates. Depletion of noradrenaline also compromises regulatory circuits. Defective regulatory T cells arise from metabolic disturbances, limiting their suppression of hyperactive effector T cells, B cells and macrophages. Failed regulation allows loss of tolerance.

Skewed T Cell Polarization

Dyslipidemia and hyperketonemia skew naïve CD4+ T cell differentiation towards pro-inflammatory Th1 and Th17 cells through mTOR and adipokine signaling. These subsets are often self-reactive due to escape of tolerance checkpoints during disrupted priming in inflamed lymphoid tissues. Regulatory T cells expressing FoxP3 are relatively underrepresented.

Hyperstimulation of Adaptive Immunity

Through bystander activation in drained lymph nodes, persistent self-antigen presentation expands self-reactive T and B cell clones over decades. This promotes emergence of effector and memory populations directed against tissues normally shielded from immunity.

Breach of Self-Tolerance

The accumulation of genetic susceptibilities, chronic priming, disrupted regulation and skewed polarization coalesce to breach checkpoint mechanisms of self-tolerance in susceptible individuals over prolonged exposures to inflammatory triggers.

Self-Perpetuating Autoimmunity

Once initiated by molecular mimicry or cryptic determinants, autoimmune attacks exacerbate tissue destruction through inflammatory mediators. This further exposes sequestered antigens fueling pathogenic adaptive immunity in a self-sustaining cascade.

Gut-Joint Axis in Inflammation

The gut-joint axis describes the important interconnected relationship between gastrointestinal tract dysfunction and rheumatoid arthritis activity. Dysbiosis caused by intestinal epithelial barrier defects, antibiotic use, infections or diet allow enteric commensal bacterial fragments like LPS to translocate from the gut lumen into circulation, promoting systemic inflammation.

Microbial mimicry between antigens on digestive pathogens and joint tissues may moreover prime cross-reactive T cell responses against joint structures over time. Evidence suggests intestinal dysbiosis and its metabolic byproducts critically drive extra-articular inflammatory manifestations in RA through mechanisms linked to chronic innate and adaptive immune stimulation.

1.4. THE IMPORTANCE OF GUT HEAL

The gastrointestinal tract plays a critical yet underappreciated role in regulating immune homeostasis and metabolic well-being. Encompassing the digestive system from mouth to anus, the gut interacts extensively with the external environment through consumption of nutrients, fluids and microbiota. This section explores the gut-immune axis and why maintaining gut health has profound implications for preventing chronic disease onset, especially autoimmunity.

The Gut Ecosystem

Over 100 trillion symbiotic microbes comprising thousands of bacterial species inhabit the gastrointestinal tract. Together with Paneth cells, antimicrobial peptides and secretory IgA antibodies, a complex ecosystem establishes colonization resistance against potential pathogens. The gut microbiota is crucial for extracting nutrients, producing vitamins, fermenting fibers, regulating inflammation and mucosal barrier integrity.

Genetics, mode of birth, antibiotic use, lifestyle and diet shape the gut microbial community from infancy. Dysbiosis refers to detrimental shifts in bacterial composition disrupting the delicate microbiota-host balance, impairing overall gut functioning and increasing disease risk over the long run if left unaddressed.

Diet acts as a major environmental driver of dysbiosis when compromised by excessive fat, sugar, chemicals or lack of fiber intake.

The Gut-Immune Axis

The gut accounts for the majority of immune cells in the entire body concentrated within patches of lymphoid aggregates called Gut Associated Lymphoid Tissue (GALT). The intestine must walk a tightrope of selectively responding vigorously against pathogens while maintaining tolerance to innocuous food and microbial antigens Translocation of commensal bacterial fragments must also be kept under tight control.

Specialized gut dendritic cells monitor the intestinal lumen and guide tolerance induction or immune activation dependent on signals received. Regulatory T cells help curb collateral inflammatory spillover. Secretory IgA antibodies neutralize microbes while promoting microbiota stability. Tight junction proteins regulate permeability between intestinal epithelial cells to prevent luminal antigen entry into circulation.

A Leaky Gut and Autoimmunity Risk

Breakdown of the Gut Barrier

Breakdown of the gut barrier can occur through various means that compromise the integrity of the intestinal epithelial cell layer and tight junction proteins. Low-grade inflammation from an imbalanced microbiome damages the barrier over time. Toxins in the modern diet like AGEs from processed foods can also disrupt integrity. Certain infections may temporarily impair barrier function.

Systemic Exposure to Gut Contents

When the barrier is compromised, luminal contents that are normally restricted to the gut lumen can now penetrate into the underlying lamina propria and enter systemic circulation. Undigested food proteins and microbial antigens are not exposed to mucosal immune cells during healthy states and eliciting tolerance.

Priming of Mucosal Immunity

In the lamina propria, these antigens stimulate dendritic cells to prime naïve T cells. Molecular mimicry between gut and joint antigens can trigger pathogenic cross-reactive T cells over years of exposure. Bacterial translocation maintains chronic innate and adaptive immune cell activation in the gut associated lymphoid tissues (GALT).

Dysregulated Lymph Node Priming

Dysregulated priming and expansion of T cell populations in the mesenteric lymph nodes occurs away from normal tolerogenic signals. Pro-inflammatory TH1 and TH17 cells dominate over regulatory phenotypes. Loss of tolerance predisposes to autoimmunity against peripheral tissues if other factors coincide in a genetically susceptible individual.

Association with Autoimmune Diseases

Studies demonstrate permeability links between gastrointestinal inflammation, microbial dysbiosis and diverse autoimmune diseases like Type 1 Diabetes, Rheumatoid Arthritis and Multiple Sclerosis. Targeting root causes of increased gut permeability forms an important strategy for prevention strategies.

Healing Approaches for A Healthy Gut

Targeted elimination diets, prebiotics and probiotics help rebalance gut flora disrupted by pharmaceuticals, infections or an unhealthy lifestyle. Bone broths, collagen peptides, L-glutamine and zinc support gut lining repair. Herbal antioxidants like turmeric soothe inflammation. Proteolytic enzymes aid food digestion and reduce antigen load. Stress management, sleep and exercise impact gut motility and secretory functions. Fixing Dietary sources of dysbiosis and leaky Gut holds promise for improving general wellness and autoimmune disease control naturally through the gut.

Chapter 2

OVERVIEW OF THE AUTOIMMUNE PROTOCOL (AIP) DIET

―――――――――

The Autoimmune Protocol (AIP) diet is a comprehensive nutritional protocol designed to support natural healing of autoimmune diseases. As we've learned, autoimmunity arises from dysfunctional immune responses driven by chronic inflammation and molecular mimicry between environmental antigens and self-proteins. The targeted elimination aspect of the AIP aims to relieve this pathogenic immune stimulation by removing common dietary triggers associated with leaky gut and immune reactivity. Pioneered by medical researcher Dr. Amy Myers, the elimination phase calls for restricting all foods in categories like grains, legumes, dairy, nightshades, eggs, alcohol and artificial ingredients for a defined period. By eliminating these potential antigenic foods, the goal is to create an anti-inflammatory environment where the gut epithelium can repair and restore barrier integrity, allowing the immune system to reset away from autoimmune attack mode.

After full elimination, the AIP involves a reintroduction phase where individual foods are slowly reintroduced one at a time to help identify personal sensitivities. Clinical studies show the AIP alleviates symptoms of diseases such as rheumatoid arthritis, multiple sclerosis and inflammatory bowel disease when diligently followed long-term. However, commitment is needed, as rushing reintroduction risks disease flare-ups. This chapter will provide an in-depth overview of both the elimination and reintroduction phases, including guidelines, meal planning tips and supplemental support options to maximize benefits.

2.1. HOW DOES AIP WORK

The Autoimmune Protocol diet is a whole foods-based elimination diet designed to reduce systemic inflammation and promote healing of the gut and immune system. By removing commonly allergenic foods from the diet, it aims to alleviate autoimmune symptoms through targeted mechanisms. This section will examine the physiological effects of the AIP and how it works to support remission of autoimmune disease.

Reducing the Antigenic Load

The gut barrier plays a crucial role in distinguishing self from non-self. In autoimmunity, leaky gut allows dietary and microbial antigens to inappropriately access and stimulate the mucosal immune system, skewing it towards reactivity over the long run. The AIP eliminates casein from dairy, wheat gluten, legumes, eggs, nuts and nightshades - all high in potential immunogenic peptides that could perpetuate intestinal inflammation and permeability issues. Removing this antigenic load gives the gut a chance to heal without constant environmental provocation confounding the restoration process. By decreasing soluble protein antigens from food that may trigger pathogenic T cells, the level of stimulation on local immunity is diminished, favoring regulatory networks over pro-inflammatory states.

Calming Chronic Inflammation

Pro-inflammatory foods like sugar, grains and highly processed omega-6 vegetable oils promote excess cytokine release, free radical production and systemic inflammation when consumed regularly. Eliminating these ingredients on the AIP curbs innate immune activation, downregulating inflammatory pathways and restoring critical balance to pro- and anti-inflammatory mediators like IL-10, TGF-β and PGE2. This soothes chronic autoimmune flares driven by dysregulated inflammation. Adopting an anti-inflammatory nutrient profile focused on whole foods simultaneously addresses metabolic endotoxemia from the gut microbiota, limiting breeches in permeability that allow lipopolysaccharides to activate toll-like receptors and perpetuate low-grade inflammation. By damping multiple mechanisms sustaining the inflammatory milieu, clinical remission becomes increasingly supported over the long-term through dietary intervention alone.

Allowing Gut Flora Restoration

An imbalanced gut microbiome characterized by deficiencies in protective commensal species lack resilience against colonization by pathogenic bacteria. The AIP diet's emphasis on traditionally prepared nutrient-dense whole foods nourishes favourable gut flora over time through fermentable fibre and polyphenols. This supports microbiota diversity and functionality tied to tight junction reinforcement, short chain fatty acid production and mucosal immune homeostasis. As the microbiota stabilizes with preferential growth of anti-inflammatory species like Bacteroides and Firmicutes, metabolic endotoxemia is reduced, pathogenicity factors lower intestinal inflammation, and regulatory immune cell populations expand to reinforce remission. Nourishing commensal bacteria in a targeted way through elimination and reintegration helps restore intestinal symbiosis as a pillar of long-lasting remission.

Removing Dietary Triggers

Identification of Triggers

The AIP strict elimination diet removes common food groups to allow resolution of inflammation and symptoms. This helps identify any foods eliciting an aberrant immune reaction on an individual level.

Elimination Phase

Nuts, eggs, dairy, grains, legumes, nightshades, seeds and other foods are removed. Processed foods, alcohol and additives are also restricted. This "resets" impaired immunity and metabolic dysfunction.

Symptom Resolution

Eliminating reactive foods alleviates inflammation, pain and other symptoms driven by immunological food sensitivity. This confirms dietary triggers were contributing to symptom flare-ups.

Reintroduction Phase

Foods are gradually reintroduced one at a time, typically every 3 days, to observe reactions. Any foods eliciting prior symptoms are identified as personal immunological triggers.

Long-Term Management

Identified triggers are avoided long-term to minimize environmental activation of the immune system and disruption of tolerance mechanisms. This supportive diet aims to reduce modifiable contributors sustaining autoimmunity.

Targeted Approach

The AIP provides an individualized, targeted approach beyond conventional diet therapies. It helps address the underlying drivers of autoinflammation on a personalized level.

Targeting Leaky Gut & Food Sensitivities

Reducing Immunological Stimuli

By removing commonly immunoreactive food groups from the diet during the elimination phase, the AIP greatly decreases signals from dietary antigens that would otherwise continuously stimulate and prime adaptive immune cells in the gut lamina propria. This removal of stimuli allows inflammation and permeability drivers to fully resolve.

Epithelial Repair

Without ongoing antigen exposure and inflammatory cytokine signaling disturbing homeostasis, gut epithelial cells can efficiently reseal gaps in the barrier layer and repair tight junction proteins that had loosened. Immune cells in the lamina propria also undergo regulatory shifts away from pro-inflammatory phenotypes as antigen traffic subsides, further supporting repair.

Identification of Triggers

The structured food reintroduction process aids recognition of specific nutrients that may directly cause immune activation and symptoms in susceptible individuals. Reactions are closely monitored to discern dose-dependent sensitivities. Multiple reintroductions help rule out false positives from other dietary or external factors.

Support for Remission

By restricting immunoreactive foods identified through AIP, adaptive immune signals driving autoimmunity are limited long-term. This deprives systemic disease processes of a modifiable environmental factor sustaining low-grade gut inflammation and breach of tolerance. Symptom relapses are less frequent.

Diet as Management

While medications aim to suppress autoimmune pathways, the AIP diet targets upstream initiators by removing food allergens and sensitivities. This two-pronged approach addressing both causes and effects enhances chances of extended remission off medication over time.

Individualized Approach

Compared to generic diets, AIP customization to an individual's unique network of dietary triggers provides a synergistic management strategy that directly supports healing of the initial injuries fueling autoimmunity in each case.

Restoring Physiological Balance

- **Nutrient Provision:** The AIP prioritizes nutrients from whole foods to support metabolic and immune homeostasis. High intake of vitamins, minerals, antioxidants and omega-3 fats counter oxidative stress and promote resolution pathways.
- **Macronutrient Profile:** Limiting high-glycemic carbs and emphasizing healthy fats and protein optimizes hormonal and metabolic signaling away from pro-inflammatory states that induce autoinflammation.
- **Microbial Metabolism:** The diverse nutrients nourish a balanced gastrointestinal microbiota. Short-chain fatty acids and other beneficial microbial metabolites are produced to maintain epithelial integrity and modulate immunity.
- **Hormonal Regulation:** Refined macro- and micronutrient balance supports adrenal, thyroid and sex hormone production to regulate lipid profiles, oxidative balance and immune cell function throughout the body.
- **Neuroendocrine Balance:** Targeting underlying causes of dysregulation confers anti-inflammatory effects through restoring HPA axis feedback, dampening "stress" cytokines and balancing the sympathetic and parasympathetic nervous systems.

- **Resolution Cascades:** As physiological stressors subside, pro-resolving mediators like lipoxins and protectins are preferentially synthesized to actively terminate chronic inflammation and breach oral tolerance.

By addressing multisystem imbalances, the AIP shifts the biochemical terrain from a state prone to sustaining autoimmunity towards one conducive to quelling pathogenic processes.

Allowing Healing Through Nutrient-Dense Foods

- **Animal Proteins:** Grass-fed and wild-caught animal proteins deliver high bioavailable iron, B12, selenium and conjugated fatty acids to rebuild tissues and mitochondria damaged by chronic disease processes.
- **Fermentable Vegetables:** Cultured and fermented options like sauerkraut provide beneficial microbes, biotin and butyrate to nourish and protect the intestinal epithelium.
- **Healthy Fats:** Traditional fats from ghee, coconut and avocado modulate immunity as sources of MCTs, vitamin E and lauric acid instead of inflammatory seed and vegetable oils.
- **Bone Broths:** Slow-cooked stocks made from chicken and beef bones deliver gelatin, collagen and minerals to aid epithelial barrier remodeling and joint recovery processes.
- **Limited Low-Sugar Fruits:** Fruits like berries provide antioxidant polyphenols, while minimizing excess sugar impacts on inflammation.
- **Nutrient-Dense Liver:** Organ meats like liver are nutritional powerhouses to support detoxification pathways and production of new cells through adequate B vitamins, iron and copper.

These nourishing whole foods paradigm fuels metabolic and immunological healing processes required for clinical remission of autoimmune disease over the long-term.

Monitoring Symptom Resolution

As gut inflammation abates and intestinal sealing tightens over weeks on the AIP diet, symptoms gradually recede - from joint pain and stiffness to fatigue, brain fog, digestive issues and skin eruptions. Tracking resolution daily through a symptom journal or checklist provides hope, encourages perseverance and allows monitoring progress and compliance. Full freedom from symptoms experienced prior to starting AIP typically signals successful elimination of reactive foods and readiness to enter the careful reintroduction phase to pinpoint individual sensitivities through trial and observation. Most medical professionals recommend committing to the full elimination diet for at least 2-6 months to allow significant time for underlying tissue healing and immunological resetting after years of dysregulation and damage. Monitoring objective markers like inflammatory biomarkers and antibody levels over the full elimination period can further validate the impact of dietary and lifestyle changes on lowering pathological immune activation.

The Reintroduction Phase

- **Stratified Process:** Foods are reintroduced in categories from most likely tolerated to most reactive - starting with small amounts of low histamine vegetables, then fruits, gluten-free grains, legumes, dairy/eggs, nuts/seeds, nightshades and finally spices.
- **Close Monitoring:** Symptom response is observed daily during each 3 day trial to catch low-level reactions. A food journal or checklist tracks onset of musculoskeletal pain, digestive issues or other prior symptoms.
- **Precautionary Protocol:** Any positive response confirms that food must still be avoided long-term or consumed sparingly to prevent future flares. Only clearly tolerated foods are reintegrated fully.
- **Repeat Testing:** Reactions may differ depending on context, such as stress levels or unrelated illness, warranting repeat testing over time for some borderline foods.
- **Self-Management:** Pinpointing personal triggers allows personalized dietary adjustments and lifestyle planning around foods that instigate loss of remission over time without medication reliance.

By understanding reactive foods, periodic re-elimination helps manage flares and gives insight towards potential medication-sparing integrated care approaches.

2.2. PHASES OF THE AIP DIET

The Autoimmune Protocol diet follows a structured two-phase approach: an initial elimination phase lasting several months to break inflammatory cycles followed by a reintroduction phase to test individual food sensitivities. Strictly adhering to each time-based phase optimizes healing potential and equips one to self-manage their autoimmune condition long-term through targeted dietary modifications.

The Elimination Phase

Length of Elimination

Lasting 2-6 months, this extended phase is recommended to provide sufficient timeline for restoration after chronic immune dysregulation and injury. The complex processes of epithelial renewal, tight junction repair, microbiota recalibration and regulatory T cell development all require weeks to reshift the gut microenvironment. Short-changing elimination risks incomplete resolution and likely recurrence upon reintroduction. Strict adherence for the full 2-6 months maximizes chances of durable remission off prolonged dietary intervention.

Removing Antigens

By stringently eliminating dietary proteins, carbohydrates, and other compounds associated with allergic-type immune responses, gut inflammation finds no fuel. No low-level stimuli provoke adaptive cell priming, memory formation or cytokine signaling to disrupt healing. Withdrawal of numerous potential immunogens gives the best environment for repair without confusion.

Facilitating Repair

The gut finds ideal conditions to repair without ongoing provocation - tight junctions link, epithelia reseal, stem cells regenerate the barrier with no interrupting signals. Immune cells can resolve to regulatory phenotypes as antigen loads subside systemically. Microbiota shift favorably to sustain the new homeostasis.

Resetting Immunity

Withdrawal of allergenic food families resets the hyperactive adaptive response through oral tolerance re-establishment. Parameters of immune exclusion at the epithelium rebalance. Regulatory networks dominate without proinflammatory polarizing influences to interfere with resetting tolerance and barrier functions.

Targeted Support

Beyond allergenic foods, all processed, synthetic additives shown to impair mucosal health are avoided for full recovery support. Nutrient-dense whole foods deliver specialized reparative elements while limiting antagonistic compounds.

Monitoring Progress

Tracking multiple parameters of resolution supplies feedback for compliance and intervention effectiveness. Biomarkers, symptoms and quality of life shifts validate dietary therapy's ability to resolve disease triggers appropriately.

Food Removal Guidelines

- **Grains (wheat, barley, rye, oats, corn):** Contain gluten/lectins disturbing microbiota balance and barrier integrity.
- **Dairy:** Contains casein and whey proteins inducing inflammation and immune reactivity in sensitive individuals.
- **Eggs:** Egg yolk comprises phosphatidylcholine and other fat molecules triggering autoimmunity.
- **Legumes:** Soaked/sprouted lentils and peas tolerated once healed due to reduced lectins.
- **Nuts & Seeds:** Contain enzyme inhibitors, anti-nutrients and inflammation-causing fats if eaten raw. Pre-soaked nuts permitted.
- **Nightshades:** Solanaceae family includes tomatoes, potatoes, peppers, eggplant carrying salsolinol suspected of autoimmune stimulation.
- **Alcohol:** Stressful to immune and liver health through increased intestinal permeability.
- **Added Sugar & Sweeteners:** Trigger food sensitivity, gut dysbiosis, inflammation and insulin resistance.
- **Fats:** Hemp, soy, corn and canola oils comprise inflammatory omega-6 fats. Grass-fed ghee/butter favored.

Foods to Focus On

- **Animal proteins:** Chicken, turkey, beef, lamb, pork, fish, shellfish, bone broth
- **Fermented veggies:** Sauerkraut, kimchi, pickles, fermented beet, carrot sticks
- **Healthy fats:** Coconut, avocado, olive oil
- **Low-sugar fruits:** Berries, citrus, melon
- **Vegetables:** Cruciferous greens, squashes
- **Optional Dairy:** Clarified butter (ghee)

Cooking Methods

Soups and Stews

Slow cooking bone broth, meat and vegetables in soups and stews for extended durations gently predigests proteins and softens fibrous tissues. This makes nutrients more bioavailable for absorption as minerals leach from bones and connective tissue collagen breaks down into amino acids and glycine. The low-and-slow cooking method also preserves heat-labile vitamins and enzymes that may otherwise degrade with high-temperature methods.

Roasting

Roasting meats and vegetables in the oven or on an open fire technique brings out flavors through Maillard reactions and caramelization. This increases some antioxidants while avoiding damaged fats created through very high-heat pan frying or grilling. Roasting seals in moisture and nutrients compared to boiling or overcooking which leach water-soluble vitamins into the cooking liquid.

Fermentation

The process of fermenting foods with beneficial bacteria increases vitamins B and K, digestive enzymes, mineral availability and generates new compounds like conjugated fatty acids. This enhances gut and immune health through preferential growth of commensal flora and anti-inflammatory short chain fatty acid production to support mucosal integrity.

Sprouting and Soaking

Presoaking nuts, seeds, grains and legumes in warm water with vitamin C activates phytases and other enzymes to partially predigest and unlock nutrients prior to eating. This reduces antigen load and workload on the digestive system to focus on recovery and support mineral absorption to nourish tissues.

Bone Broth

Slow cooking bones releases minerals and collagen into a warm, easily absorbed liquid goldmine for gut repair and symptom relief. Joint-soothing compounds like glycosaminoglycans aid resolution of arthritic driven by chronic gut inflammation.

Symptom Management

Resolution Monitoring

Careful daily documentation of symptom scores, severity ratings, pain levels, energy/fatigue, bowel habits, skin lesions and other barometers provides quantitative data to assess response overtime. This validates effective dietary changes and determines if modification or re-elimination is needed should symptoms unexpectedly reemerge during the process.

Individual Response

While most see improvements within 2-6 months, response will vary depending on disease complexity, previous damage extent, underlying genetic factors and overall health. Those with longer duration or more severe presentations may require 6-12 months for full resolution as healing occurs gradually at both macro and microscopic levels.

Holistic Support

Targeted supplementation nourishes underlying mitochondrial function, glutathione production and Phase 1/2 detox pathways to aid the body in safely eliminating reactive metabolites and resolving inflammation. Herbal extracts and lifestyle factors further support reduction of residual symptoms.

Hope and Perseverance

Consistently noting positive shifts day by day in a symptom journal encourages commitment to healing, especially when gains seem minor. This document serves as inspiration when difficulties arise to continue naturally managing illness without dependence on uninformed quick fixes.

Guiding Reintroduction

Methodical reintroduction using food diaries establishes personalized trigger maps to avoid relapse. Should symptoms return, records guide appropriate re-elimination or modification to support long-lasting remission independent of the diet.

Self-Care and Relief

Achieving equilibrium empowers ongoing wellness through awareness of triggers and healthy adaptions. Remission signifies victory over disease's disruption of quality life, validating discipline through a whole lifestyle approach.

The Reintroduction Phase

After 6+ months on strict elimination, reintroducing foods tests tolerance to determine lifelong dietary modifications. One new potential trigger food is tested weekly to discern reaction separately from the full protocol.

Reintroduction Process

Single Food Reintroduction

Careful reintroduction of only one new food at a time, eaten in small isolated portions every 3 days, allows for accurate assessment of individual responses. This stringent approach ensures any returned symptoms can unambiguously be linked to the specific rechallenged ingredient without interference or confusion from additional variables.

Symptom Monitoring

Paying close attention to subtle signs of gastrointestinal distress, joint discomfort, skin reactions or other characteristic symptoms provides valuable feedback over the 72-hour window. Monitoring energy levels, mood and overall sense of wellness further informs reactions. A symptom diary tracks outcomes.

No Reaction Acceptance

If wellness is maintained without return of previous issues, the food can likely be reintroduced as tolerated into the long-term menu. However, it remains important to continue periodically checking for potential delayed or subtle responses initially masked by the body's resilient nature.

Should any autoimmune symptoms resurface promptly after a single food reintroduction, that ingredient is clearly identified as a trigger to avoid long-term. The body's message should be respected for ongoing management of underlying dysregulation and prevention of relapse.

Order of Difficulty

Reintroducing the most challenging food families like legumes first due to failure of previous tolerance provides the hardest test cases upfront. Easier categories are left for later should issues arise from initial harder reintroductions requiring more elimination time.

Additional Re-Elimination

If multiple reactive foods appear together upon reintroduction, the full elimination protocol may need revisiting longer to allow deeper resolution before again attempting to remap trigger foods through cautious rechallenging.

Developing Maintenance

An individualized lifelong management strategy is key to living well without dependence on the diet long-term. Careful self-awareness and professional guidance help balance wellness, quality of life, and disease control goals over the long haul.

This gradual process identifies specific food sensitivities and intolerances for tailored dietary care. Knowing triggers empowers informed choices around social eating and lifestyle factors impacting wellness long-term. Together, the targeted removal and reintroduction plan offers a comprehensive system for resetting immunity.

Ongoing Commitment

Autoimmune conditions frequently necessitate continuous vigilance against underlying triggers that fuel pathogenic immune processes over decades. While remission indicates clinical resolution, residual immunological dysregulation persists susceptible to reactivation. Strategic re-elimination cycles reinforce regulatory networks by periodically reassessing elimination fundamentals under a functional medicine provider. This accounts for shifting environmental exposures and biological changes with aging, fortifying individualized protocols long-term.

Stress-reducing practices, restorative sleep, nutrient-dense menus, targeted supplementation and regular exercise further strengthen natural resistance against stressors perturbing homeostasis. Periodic reassessment couples with holistic self-care supporting the intricate balance between genetics and environment. Adhering to personalized anti-inflammatory nutrition, toxin avoidance, mental well-being and physical activity forms the foundation for stabilizing health autonomy and preventing flare recurrence through lifelong adaptive strategies. Long-term preservation of remission quality requires commitment to this comprehensive lifestyle approach.

2.3. HOW DOES AIP SUPPORT AUTOIMMUNE HEALTH

The Autoimmune Protocol diet is designed from the ground up to counter pathogenic factors sustaining autoimmunity. By targeting gut integrity, microbiome balance, systemic inflammation and dietary triggers through strategic whole foods elimination and reintroduction, it aims to alleviate autoimmune disease activity naturally over time. This section explores the multifaceted mechanisms by which AIP nourishes remission.

Mending the Leaky Gut

Impaired Barrier Function

Compromised intestinal epithelial barrier function is a key driver of autoimmunity, allowing undigested antigens and toxins to translocate into tissues where they provoke inflammation. The gut lining plays a crucial role in containment.

Targeted Nourishment

AIP elimination and foods like bone broths, fermented foods, and nutrient-dense whole produce directly nourish and support renewal of intestinal cells. Specific amino acids, collagen peptides, fatty acids and antioxidants aid renewal of cellular junctions that form a semi-permeable barrier.

Reducing Inflammatory Load

Strategic removal of common antigenic triggers reduces surface inflammation in the gut, allowing optimal conditions for epithelial repair and sealing of tight junctions between cells. This restores barrier selectivity and cuts off stimulation of immunopathology.

Healing Provisions

The array of targeted gut-supportive nutrients in the AIP arsenal effectively "patches holes" in the intestinal wall that had facilitated translocation of reactive substances into tissues, thereby countering the root driver of autoimmune dysregulation.

Barrier Integrity Restored

Re-establishing proper barrier function through elimination and focused enteral nutrition forms the cornerstone of autoimmune resolution by depriving dysregulated immunity of its provocative fuel and environment for chronic activation.

Rebalancing the Microbiome

Microbiota Composition

A balanced gut microbiota comprising diverse commensal flora conferring metabolic and immune benefits becomes displaced by opportunistic pathogens during dysbiosis. This disrupts innate immune homeostasis.

Prebiotic Provision

AIP nourishes beneficial bacterial populations through an abundance of fermentable fiber from vegetables, resistant starches and non-starch polysaccharides generating short-chain fatty acids as preferred flora fuels.

Eliminating Dysbiotic Factors

Restricting refined carbohydrates, industrial seed and vegetable oils depletes commensals while promoting dysbiotic pathogens and inflammatory metabolites like LPS. Their removal allows preferential regrowth of a healthier profile.

Tight Junction Fortification

Butyrate and other SCFA end-products of fiber fermentation by commensals support epithelial integrity and robust tight junctions, restricting pathogenic bacterial interaction with the intestinal lining.

Metabolic Control

A diversified microbiota composition confers optimal intestinal regulation over dysbiotic metabolites including reactive oxygen species, amines and enzymatic activity influencing autoimmune risk factor expression locally and systemically.

Taming Systemic Inflammation

Chronic inflammation endangers normal physiological functioning and sustains autoimmune pathology. AIP calms inflammation through careful macronutrient ratios focussed on protein and healthy fats with limited carbohydrates to prevent glycemic variability, insulin resistance and associated pro-inflammatory effects. Emphasis on anti-inflammatory spices, coloring phytonutrients from plant foods and elimination of processed omega-6 sources further quenches pathogenic inflammatory pathways centrally involved in autoimmunity expression.

Optimizing Nutrient Status

Nutrient Reservoirs

To withstand environmental insults and restore immunological equilibrium, ample stores of cofactors supporting phase I/II detoxification, antioxidation, methylation and more must replenish depleted levels from chronic illness and an SAD diet lacking density.

Anti-Inflammatory Provision

AIP menus emphasize nutrient powerhouses like fatty fish and organ meats, fermented foods, leafy greens and non-starchy vegetables providing the raw materials for biosynthesis of glutathione, NO, COX inhibitors and resolving counteracting metabolic inflammation.

Restoring Metabolic Capacity

Micronutrients coax genetic expression and enzymatic activity back to healthy homeostatic set-points, recalibrating regulatory networks controlling immune cell differentiation and effector functions to resolve from a dysregulated state.

Physiological Resiliency

With deficits addressed, natural defenses against environmental insults regain integrity, reinforced by elimination of reactive exposures that can overwhelm even optimized physiology in autoimmune-susceptible individuals with imperfect tolerance mechanisms.

Foundations for Healing

This focus on nutrient-dense traditional whole foods establishes the necessary biochemical infrastructure and substrates for physiological systems to marshal restorative processes, supported by simultaneous antigen avoidance, leading to clinical remission over time.

Addressing Detoxification

The liver plays a critical role in metabolizing and clearing reactive compounds that can challenge immunity and homeostasis if not properly detoxified. However, chronic illness and environmental exposures can overwhelm and weaken the liver's phases I and II detox pathways over time. AIP emphasizes nutrient-dense green vegetables, herbs, spices and cruciferous foods like broccoli and cauliflower that support these phases through stimulating production of antioxidants and metabolizing enzymes. Staying well-hydrated and prioritizing rest further aids the liver in safely transforming and excreting exogenous compounds. Optimizing detoxification in this way lessens the toxic burden on the body that can contribute to low-grade inflammation and autoimmune stimulation. Supporting optimal liver function through focused nutritional and lifestyle interventions therefore serves as an important part of the holistic AIP approach to gaining terrain dominance over pathogenic triggers.

Managing Stress Factors

Glucocorticoid Balance

Chronic stress dysregulates the hypothalamic-pituitary-adrenal (HPA) axis, resulting in prolonged elevated or insufficient cortisol levels that fuel systemic inflammation and compromise intestinal barrier integrity. AIP supports normalization of the HPA axis and glucocorticoid signaling through elimination of reactive foods and incorporation of plant-based fats, fermented foods and nutrients like B vitamins, which help moderate stress responses and promote balanced adrenal function over time.

Calming Influences

The short and medium chain fatty acids from coconut oil have been shown to stimulate production of ketone bodies when metabolized, which can promote relaxation while also supporting focus and cognition. Additionally, coconut oil is rich in tryptophan, an amino acid precursor to serotonin that helps regulate mood and anxiety levels. Consuming these anti-anxiety nutrients as part of AIP can help offset mental stress.

Relaxation Techniques

Mind-body practices like yoga and meditation train the body's relaxation response, counteracting symptoms of stress like elevated inflammation, disrupted digestion and disturbed sleep patterns. Making time for adequate, high-quality rest also allows the mind and body to recharge effectively. Incorporating these relaxation techniques regularly supports overall mental wellness, gut health and healing on AIP.

Social Reinforcements

Sharing experiences with a supportive community provides accountability advantages that can help sustain lifestyle changes long-term. Additionally, prioritizing meaningful social connections and leisurely activities shown to buffer stress levels complements AIP goals of reducing compounding mental pressures that exacerbate autoimmune conditions.

Alleviating Compounding Stressors

Implementing a multifaceted approach addressing social, dietary, mental and physical aspects of the holistic lifestyle aims to alleviate glucocorticoid dysregulation and numerous other mechanisms by which psychological stress can exacerbate autoimmune pathology over time. Relieving these compounding influences supports optimal healing results.

In essence, AIP addresses root drivers with a multi-targeted nutritional intervention emphasizing gut repair, immunoregulation, metabolic control and identification of personal triggers to progressively bring autoimmune conditions into remission from the inside out through whole foods focused elimination and reintroduction over weeks and months.

2.3.1. Immune Regulation

A delicate balance between tolerance and protective immunity against pathogens underlies health. In autoimmunity, dysregulated immune responses actively promote chronic destruction. The AIP diet supports restoration of the immune system's natural regulatory capacity through targeted mechanisms.

Calming Inflammatory Cytokines

Excess pro-inflammatory cytokines like TNF-α, IL-1β and IL-6 characterize autoimmune inflammatory milieu. AIP calms overactive cytokine signaling through omega-3 polyunsaturated fatty acids from fish and use of spices with cytokine modulating properties. Additionally, removing aggravating foods during elimination and reintroduction reduces innate and adaptive immune stimulation that intensifies pathogenic cytokine production over the long term.

Balancing T Helper Cell Subsets

Imbalances between Th1, Th2, Th17 and regulatory T cell populations perturb immune homeostasis. AIP nourishes a balanced T cell phenotype conducive to tolerance through prebiotic fiber encouraging Treg promotion, vitamin D from fat fish and nutrient density avoiding T cell polarizing deficiencies that skew responses away from tolerance. Together, these mechanisms support controlled, context-appropriate immunity.

Optimizing Regulatory T Cells

Tregs dampen autoimmune inflammatory cascades, preventing inappropriate autoimmunity. Fermentable fibers, vitamin A from organ meats and antioxidants in AIP fruits/veggies fuel Treg proliferation, suppressive IL-10/TGF-β cytokine release and trafficking ability to resolve tissue inflammation and replenish self-tolerance lost in autoimmune conditions over the long run.

Strengthening Epithelial Barriers

Intestinal permeability drives breaking of self-tolerance. AIP mends leaky gut by supplying collagen precursors like gelatin and MCTs for epithelial barrier fortification through tight junction reinforcement and reduction of surface inflammatory signals that disrupt junctional proteins and increase permeability defects. This insulates immunity from inappropriate self-antigen exposures over time.

Supporting Regulatory B Cells

When activated appropriately, Bregs suppress T cell-mediated autoimmunity and promote tolerance induction. Fermented foods in AIP nourish the microbiota for short-chain fatty acid regulation of Breg functions like IL-10 production that downmodulate inflammatory Th17 responses, quenching autoimmune pathogenicity at its source through restoration of lost regulatory balance.

Addressing Nutritional Deficiencies

Micronutrient insufficiencies impair regulatory immune functions. AIP focuses on nutrient-dense whole foods to optimize intake of vitamins A, D, E, B6, folate and minerals like zinc, copper and selenium instrumental for Treg development and suppressive capacity, enzymatic antioxidant protection, epithelial barrier integrity and metabolic processes that maintain immune balance. This biochemical foundation supports restoration of lost tolerance over time.

Optimizing Gut-Immune Crosstalk

Chronic dysbiosis impairs the gut-lymph signaling axis. AIP enriches beneficial microbial fermenters through prebiotic-rich vegetables and reductions in dysbiosis-promoting sugars and pro-inflammatory omega-6 oils. Prebiotics stimulate short-chain fatty acid regulators of Treg differentiation in the intestinal immune system interface. Meanwhile, eliminating reactivity-triggering foods allows restoration of gut mucosal immune quiescence through direct receptor-mediated tolerogenic signals devoid of ongoing antigenic stimulation—strengthening epithelial homeostatic immunity and maintenance of the balanced intestinal immune phenotype.

Reducing Metabolic Stress

Chronic stress contributes to maladaptive immune polarization. AIP focuses on nutrients like vitamins B1, B5, magnesium and healthy fats that aid energy production and balance cortisol, promoting relaxation through reduction of aggravating foods and lifestyle habits empowering stress resilience. This counters glucocorticoid dysregulation and metabolic endotoxemia perpetuating autoimmunity, supporting a physiological milieu where tolerance and regulatory responses prevail once more.

2.3.2. Gut Health Benefits

The gut microbiota and intestinal barrier integrity hold pivotal roles in autoimmune pathogenesis. AIP targets restoration of optimal gut function and environment through foundational support of the microbiome ecology and GI mucosal defenses.

Nourishing Beneficial Bacteria

Prebiotic-rich vegetables encouraged by AIP act as preferred fuel for microbiota symbionts promoting regulatory immunity and barrier protection. This supports diversity and metabolic capacity tied to short-chain fatty acid production lowering pH and offering epithelial protection against inflammation-inducing toxins. Individualized elimination and reintroduction further identifies foods supporting dysbiosis to avoid ongoing imbalances.

Strengthening Intestinal Barrier Integrity

Nutrients in AIP foods like zinc, vitamin A, and collagen-containing gelatin from bone broth directly reinforce tight junction proteins maintaining intestinal barrier function weakened in autoimmunity. Fermented options stimulate tight junction remodeling genes. Removal of antigenic foods reduces oxidative stress and inflammatory signals disrupting barrier architecture to allow repair in a nutrient-sufficient environment tailored for healing.

Balancing pH and Microbial Metabolism

Focus on non-starchy vegetables and exclusion of pro-dysbiosis sugars/grains maintains a neutral colonic pH favoring commensal proliferation and production of short-chain fatty acids like butyrate exerting anti-inflammatory effects throughout the gut and systemically. This balances luminal biochemical environment dysregulated in autoimmunity.

Supporting Mucus Layer Integrity

Fermented foods stimulate mucin-producing goblet cells forming a protective mucus layer of defense. Protein-rich AIP nourishes this to buffer the epithelium from noxious antigens, pathogenic adherence/toxicity that would otherwise disrupt tight junctions in a compromised mucus barrier state often seen in autoimmune conditions.

Managing Pathogenic Microbes

Prebiotic fibers selective nourish protective flora to outcompete pathogenic microbes associated with leaky gut and systemic inflammation. Removal of reactive foods disrupts favorable conditions for opportunists dysregulated in autoimmunity through targeted nutrient interventions emphasizing fermented options like sauerkraut for ongoing balance support once achieved.

Reducing Toxins and Allergens

By avoiding heavily sprayed non-organic fruits and vegetables as well as dairy, eggs and other potential allergens during elimination and identifying triggers post-reintroduction, AIP limits allergen and environmental toxin exposure that can compromise gut barrier integrity. This reduces inflammatory signals exacerbating autoimmunity over the long term.

Supporting Detoxification Capacity

AIP plant compounds from cruciferous vegetables, berries and caffeic acid-rich coffee substitutes aid Phase I/II liver detox pathways handling gut-derived toxins able to disturb systemic immunity if accumulated. Nutrient cofactors like B vitamins, selenium and glutathione further bolster hepatic clearance weakened under autoimmune inflammatory duress, lessening pathogenic stimuli.

Optimizing Digestive Health

Focus on traditionally-prepared whole foods, bone broth for digestive enzymes and probiotic/prebiotic pairing supports robust gastrointestinal motility, secretions and transit tied to immune tolerance induction via epithelial sampling of luminal contents. Daily fiber aids regular bowel movements, easing constipation and small intestinal bacterial overgrowth linked to autoimmunity. Gentle exercise furtherance peristalsis without compromising recovery. Together these optimize assimilatory function disrupted in autoimmune dysfunction.

2.4. RECOMMENDED SUPPLEMENTS TO SUPPORT HEALING

While whole foods are the foundation, certain supplements address micronutrient needs and recovery on the biochemical level. These research-backed adjuncts support AIP when used judiciously under medical guidance.

Omega-3 Fatty Acids

The long-chain omega-3 fatty acids EPA and DHA play a significant role in resolving inflammation and maintaining optimal immune cell function. As precursors to potent resolvins and protectins, daily intake of 1-3 grams through fatty fish, fish oil, or algal oil supplements helps counterbalance the pro-inflammatory omega-6 fatty acids that are often elevated in autoimmune disorders. EPA and DHA act to calm endothelial activation, regulate cytokine signaling cascades, and reduce production of reactive oxygen species that accelerate tissue damage over time. Krill oil, with its enhanced astaxanthin content, provides excellent stability to the fragile omega-3s as they undergo metabolic processing, further protecting cells from oxidative damage. Incorporating omega-3s as targeted anti-inflammatory messengers is therefore a key facet of the AIP approach, supporting resolution of chronic inflammation at the root of autoimmune pathology.

Vitamin D3

This steroid hormone plays a vital role in maintaining immune tolerance, gut barrier function and microbiota composition. However, deficiency is highly correlated with autoimmune disease prevalence due to insufficient sun exposure and dietary intake. Supplementing with 5,000-10,000 IU per day works to elevate 25-hydroxy vitamin D serum levels into the protective range of 40-60 ng/ml, supporting Treg population balance, cellular differentiation and calcium/bone homeostasis. Taking vitamin D3 alongside vitamin K2 aids absorption, while moderate sun exposure also helps boost levels naturally. Addressing insufficiency through these targeted means constitutes an important component of the AIP framework for restoring immunological equilibrium.

Curcumin

A principal active compound in turmeric, curcumin has potent anti-inflammatory properties stemming from its ability to downregulate the NF-kB and AP-1 transcription factor complexes that drive expression of many pro-inflammatory genes. Through inhibition of COX-2, 5-LOX and other enzymes, curcumin reduces biosynthesis of inflammatory eicosanoids, cytokines and reactive oxygen species that promote tissue damage. Clinical studies have found doses of 500-1000mg per day can help resolve inflammation by aiding regulatory T cell modulation and the restoration of immune tolerance at inflamed sites. Curcumin is highly fat-soluble, so consuming it with piperine from black pepper can boost absorption and bioavailability substantially to maximize its systemic benefits within the AIP framework.

Vitamin B Complex

Optimal functioning of crucial metabolic processes like methylation cycling, mitochondrial energy production from carbohydrate/fat burning, neurotransmitter synthesis and immune modulation relies on sufficient intake and balanced status of all B vitamins. However, autoimmune conditions can compromise absorptive capacity and increase metabolic demand. A high-potency, broad-spectrum B complex supplement delivers the array of water and fat-soluble B vitamins required to reinforce depleted cellular foundations. When possible, using methylated forms ensures maximal uptake and intracellular activation especially for those with genetic variants attenuating traditional B vitamin utilization. Addressing imbalances restores numerous core physiological functions disrupted in autoimmunity.

Vitamin C

As a primary water-soluble antioxidant, vitamin C defenses physiological systems from damage by reactive oxidative metabolites known to drive pathogenic inflammation. However, its levels deplete rapidly under conditions of elevated oxidative load. Supplemental intakes of 1000-2000mg per day divided throughout the day go beyond customary Recommended Dietary Allowances insufficient to offset oxidative burdens experienced with autoimmune dysfunction. The resulting super-physiological concentrations facilitate roles in collagen production, neutrophil and T cell immunity critical to maintaining connective tissue integrity, blood vessel flexibility and epithelial barrier repair integral to recovery processes. Supporting optimal Vitamin C status thus reinforces numerous protective functions compromised in autoimmunity.

Probiotics

Reinstating a healthy balance of commensal microbes aligns the gut ecosystem, supporting restoration of intestinal barrier function and regulated systemic immunity. Careful selection and therapeutic dosing of beneficial bacteria, such as Lactobacillus rhamnosus GG, Bifidobacterium lactis Bl-04 and the yeast Saccharomyces boulardii, confer these advantages by competitively inhibiting pathogenic overgrowth while stimulating robust bile acid metabolism and anti-inflammatory Treg responses through pattern recognition receptor signaling. Clinical trials find consuming 5-10 billion CFUs per day from various strains provides the resilience-building effects. However, these benefits optimize once gut tolerance and dysbiosis remedies through the removal of immunological triggers and optimized nutrition allow probiotic colonies to durably engraft later in the AIP framework as intestinal health reconstitutes fully.

Bone Broth Concentrates

Rich, homemade bone broth simmered for extended periods infuses a complex matrix of wound-healing and gut-protective nutrients into an easily digestible whole food. Sipping bone broth supplies bioavailable collagen peptides, glycine and glutamine plus calcium, magnesium and other minerals to rebuild intestinal lining and joint structures compromised by autoimmunity. For individuals short on time for true bone broth preparation, supplemental collagen peptides provide similar foundational support in concentrated doses of 5-10 grams daily. These foundational building blocks reinforce gastrointestinal permeability, encourage satiety hormone release and strengthen weakened connective tissues from a natural anti-inflammatory source integral to AIP recovery objectives focused on mucosal and systemic restoration.

Prescription Omega-3s

For individuals facing debilitating autoimmune complications where standard doses of dietary and supplemental omega-3s prove insufficient, closely monitored adjunct therapy with prescription formulations can provide a targeted boost. Triglyceride products delivering doses exceeding 1-2 grams per day of EPA and DHA through higher absorption formulations achieve physiologically active concentrations with longer half-lives ideal for resolving severe inflammation. Brands like Lovaza and Vascepa contain highly concentrated omega-3s as ethyl esters or re-esterified triglycerides that bypass digestive breakdown for increased delivery to tissues. When taken under medical guidance as part of a comprehensive treatment program combining prescription support, optimized nutrition and lifestyle practices, these potent prescription options offer amplified anti-inflammatory effects to address highly active autoimmune disease better than over-the-counter sources alone.

Chapter 3

COMPREHENSIVE FOOD LIST

This chapter will comprehensively outline the foods that are compliant with the Autoimmune Protocol diet. Knowing which ingredients are acceptable according to each phase of the program is integral for achieving healing success. The elimination phase focuses on easily digestible proteins, non-starchy vegetables, healthy fats and limited fruits. Bone broth also plays an important role in this phase for its gut-healing properties. Foods like meat, seafood, eggs, coconut products and avocados provide nourishment while strictly removing common triggers.

As one progresses to the reintroduction phase after a minimum of 6 months on the full elimination, structured guidance is needed. This chapter will break down the specific grains, nuts, seeds, nightshades and eggs that may be tested individually for tolerance once the baseline healing has occurred. Careful reintroduction relies on clarity around timing and food categories to properly identify personal sensitivities. With support, optimizing whole food nutrient intake targets the root causes of inflammation and gastrointestinal impairment.

Comprehensive food lists in this chapter synthesize AIP compliance according to important considerations like macronutrients, micronutrients and preparation methods. Referring back to these guidelines builds confidence in meal planning and long-term protocol navigation. The goal is empowering self-management of autoimmune health through informed, targeted whole food selections as well as avoidance of revealed triggers. This detailed resource aims to properly equip individuals for reversal success utilizing the full potential of the AIP framework.

3.1. AIP-APPROVED FOODS

Organ Meat and Offal

Organ meats, also known as offal, are a cornerstone of the AIP diet due to their exceptional nutrient density. These include:

- Liver
- Heart
- Kidneys
- Sweetbreads
- Tongue

The AIP diet recommends incorporating organ meats at least five times a week. These foods are powerhouses of essential nutrients, including:

- Vitamins A, D, E, and K
- B-complex vitamins, especially B12
- Essential fatty acids
- Minerals like iron, zinc, and selenium

Organ meats support immune function, reduce inflammation, and promote overall health. They can significantly improve energy levels and aid detoxification processes. For those new to organ meats, starting with milder options like heart or tongue may be more palatable. Liver, while highly nutritious, has a stronger flavor and can be incorporated into ground meat dishes or pâtés. It's important to source organ meats from high-quality, preferably grass-fed or pasture-raised animals to maximize nutrient content and minimize exposure to toxins.

Fish and Shellfish

The AIP diet strongly emphasizes the consumption of fish and shellfish, recommending at least three servings per week. Wild-caught varieties are preferred, but sustainably farmed options are acceptable alternatives.

Key benefits of fish and shellfish include:

- Rich source of omega-3 fatty acids (EPA and DHA)
- High-quality, easily digestible protein
- Essential minerals like iodine and selenium
- Natural source of vitamin D

Fish particularly high in omega-3s include:

- Salmon
- Mackerel
- Sardines
- Anchovies
- Herring

Shellfish, such as oysters, mussels, and clams, are nutrient powerhouses, offering concentrated amounts of zinc, iron, and B12. The anti-inflammatory properties of omega-3s in fish and shellfish support heart health, brain function, and immune regulation. They also play a crucial role in managing autoimmune conditions by reducing systemic inflammation. When selecting fish, be mindful of mercury content, opting for smaller fish species more frequently. For those concerned about sustainability, resources like the Monterey Bay Aquarium's Seafood Watch can guide choices.

Vegetables of All Kinds

A diverse and abundant intake of vegetables is crucial in the AIP diet, with a recommendation of at least eight servings daily. This emphasis on vegetable consumption ensures a wide range of phytonutrients, vitamins, and minerals essential for overall health and managing autoimmune conditions.

Key benefits of a vegetable-rich diet include:

- High fiber content for gut health
- Antioxidants to combat oxidative stress
- Essential vitamins and minerals
- Phytonutrients with anti-inflammatory properties

Vegetables to focus on:

- Leafy greens (spinach, kale, collards)
- Cruciferous vegetables (broccoli, cauliflower, Brussels sprouts)

- Root vegetables (sweet potatoes, carrots, beets)
- Squashes (butternut, acorn, zucchini)
- Alliums (onions, garlic, leeks)

To maximize nutrient intake, aim for a variety of colors and types of vegetables. Cooking methods can affect nutrient availability; for instance, lightly steaming cruciferous vegetables can enhance their digestibility while preserving nutrients. Rotating vegetables seasonally can provide a broader spectrum of nutrients and support local, sustainable agriculture. Consider incorporating lesser-known vegetables like kohlrabi, celeriac, or different varieties of radishes to expand your nutrient profile and culinary experiences.

Leafy Green Vegetables

Leafy green vegetables are a vital component of the AIP diet, offering a concentrated source of nutrients with minimal calories. They provide an array of vitamins, minerals, and phytonutrients that support various bodily functions and help manage autoimmune conditions.

Key nutrients found in leafy greens:

- Vitamin A (as beta-carotene)
- Vitamin C
- Vitamin K
- Folate
- Calcium
- Magnesium
- Iron

Popular leafy greens in the AIP diet include:

- Spinach
- Kale
- Collard greens
- Swiss chard
- Arugula
- Mustard greens
- Watercress

These vegetables support bone health, immune function, and energy production. They also contain compounds that aid in detoxification processes and have anti-inflammatory properties. To maximize nutrient absorption, consider pairing leafy greens with a source of healthy fat, as some nutrients are fat-soluble. Rotating different types of leafy greens can ensure a broader range of nutrients and prevent overconsumption of any potentially problematic compounds. For those with thyroid issues, it's important to note that raw cruciferous leafy greens contain goitrogens, which can interfere with thyroid function if consumed in large amounts. Lightly cooking these greens can reduce their goitrogenic properties.

Colorful Vegetables and Fruit

The AIP diet emphasizes consuming a rainbow of colorful vegetables and fruits to ensure a diverse range of antioxidants and phytonutrients. Each color group offers unique health benefits and supports different aspects of immune function and overall health.

Color groups and their benefits:

- Red (e.g., beets, strawberries): Rich in lycopene and anthocyanins, supporting heart health and reducing inflammation.
- Purple/Blue (e.g., blueberries, eggplant): High in resveratrol and flavonoids, offering neuroprotective and anti-aging benefits.
- Yellow/Orange (e.g., sweet potatoes, apricots): Abundant in beta-carotene and vitamin C, supporting eye health and immune function.
- Green (e.g., broccoli, kiwi): Packed with chlorophyll and lutein, aiding in detoxification and eye health.
- White (e.g., cauliflower, pears): Contain allicin and quercetin, supporting heart health and immune function.

When incorporating fruits, it's important to monitor fructose intake, aiming for 10-40g daily, with 20g being optimal. This approach helps manage blood sugar levels while still benefiting from the essential vitamins, minerals, and antioxidants in fruits. Berries are particularly recommended due to their low sugar content and high antioxidant properties. Rotating seasonal produce can ensure a varied nutrient intake and support local agriculture. Remember that while fruits offer numerous health benefits, they should be consumed in moderation as part of a balanced AIP diet.

Cruciferous Vegetables

Cruciferous vegetables are a standout category in the AIP diet, known for their potent health-promoting properties. These vegetables belong to the Brassicaceae family and are rich in fiber, vitamins, minerals, and unique sulfur-containing compounds called glucosinolates.

Key cruciferous vegetables include:

- Broccoli and broccolini
- Cauliflower
- Brussels sprouts
- Cabbage (all varieties)
- Kale and collard greens
- Bok choy
- Arugula
- Radishes
- Turnips and rutabaga

The health benefits of cruciferous vegetables are numerous:

- Support detoxification processes in the body
- Possess anti-inflammatory properties
- May have anti-cancer effects due to compounds like sulforaphane
- Rich in fiber, supporting gut health and digestion
- High in vitamin C, K, and folate

While incredibly nutritious, it's important to note that cruciferous vegetables contain goitrogens, which can interfere with thyroid function if consumed in large quantities, especially when raw. For individuals with thyroid issues, lightly cooking these vegetables can reduce their goitrogenic properties. Fermented cruciferous vegetables, like sauerkraut or kimchi (without non-AIP ingredients), can offer additional probiotic benefits while potentially reducing goitrogenic effects.

Roots, Tubers, and Winter Squash

Roots, tubers, and winter squash are essential components of the AIP diet, providing complex carbohydrates, fiber, and a wealth of nutrients. These foods offer sustained energy and support gut health, making them valuable for those managing autoimmune conditions.

Key examples include:

- Sweet potatoes
- Cassava (yuca)
- Taro
- Parsnips

- Beets
- Carrots
- Turnips
- Rutabaga
- Winter squash varieties (acorn, butternut, kabocha, pumpkin)

These foods are rich in:

- Complex carbohydrates for sustained energy
- Dietary fiber for gut health
- Beta-carotene (precursor to vitamin A)
- Potassium for heart and muscle function
- Antioxidants and other phytonutrients

Roots, tubers, and winter squash can be prepared in various ways, including roasting, steaming, or mashing. They can serve as excellent replacements for grains in many dishes. For example, spiralized zucchini or spaghetti squash can replace pasta, while mashed cauliflower can substitute for mashed potatoes. When consuming these foods, be mindful of your individual carbohydrate tolerance and adjust portions accordingly. Fermenting some root vegetables, like beets, can enhance their digestibility and provide probiotic benefits.

Onion Family (Alliums)

The onion family, scientifically known as Alliums, plays a crucial role in the AIP diet due to their flavor-enhancing properties and numerous health benefits. These vegetables are known for their distinct sulfur-containing compounds, which contribute to their pungent aroma and taste.

Key members of the Allium family include:

- Onions (all varieties)
- Garlic
- Leeks
- Shallots
- Chives
- Scallions (green onions)
- Ramps (wild leeks)

Health benefits of Alliums:

- Rich in organosulfur compounds with antimicrobial properties
- Support cardiovascular health by helping to lower blood pressure and cholesterol
- Boost immune function
- Possess anti-inflammatory properties
- May have anticancer effects

Alliums are versatile in cooking and can be used raw, sautéed, roasted, or in soups and stews. They add depth of flavor to dishes without the need for non-AIP compliant seasonings. Garlic, in particular, is known for its potent medicinal properties and can be consumed in various forms, including raw, cooked, or as infused oil. When using onions and garlic, allowing them to sit for a few minutes after chopping can enhance their beneficial compounds. For those sensitive to FODMAPs, cooking alliums thoroughly or using infused oils can help reduce potential digestive discomfort while still providing flavor and some health benefits.

Sea Vegetables

Sea vegetables, also known as seaweed, are highly nutritious additions to the AIP diet. These marine plants are rich in minerals and unique compounds not commonly found in land vegetables. However, it's important to note that immune-stimulating algae like chlorella and spirulina are typically excluded from the AIP diet.

Common sea vegetables include:

- Nori (used in sushi wraps)
- Kombu
- Wakame
- Dulse
- Arame
- Hijiki

Key benefits of sea vegetables:

- Excellent source of iodine, crucial for thyroid function
- Rich in minerals like iron, calcium, and magnesium
- Contain unique antioxidants like fucoxanthin
- Provide dietary fiber, including some prebiotic fibers
- Source of omega-3 fatty acids (in smaller amounts)

Sea vegetables can be incorporated into the diet in various ways:

- As wraps for sushi-style rolls
- Added to soups and stews (especially kombu for flavor and nutrients)
- Sprinkled as flakes over salads or other dishes
- Used to make broths

When consuming sea vegetables, it's important to be mindful of their high iodine content, especially for those with thyroid conditions. Start with small amounts and increase gradually. Also, be aware of potential contamination with heavy metals and choose sea vegetables from reputable sources. Some people may prefer to soak and rinse sea vegetables before use to reduce sodium content. Incorporating a variety of sea vegetables can provide a broad spectrum of nutrients and flavors to enhance the AIP diet.

Mushrooms

Mushrooms are a unique and valuable component of the AIP diet, offering a range of health benefits and adding depth to meals. As edible fungi, they provide a distinct nutritional profile compared to plants and animals.

Common edible mushrooms include:

- White button mushrooms
- Cremini (baby bella)
- Portobello
- Shiitake
- Oyster
- Maitake (hen of the woods)
- Lion's mane
- Reishi (typically used medicinally)

Health benefits of mushrooms:

- Rich in B vitamins, especially niacin and riboflavin
- Good source of selenium, an important antioxidant mineral
- Contain beta-glucans, which support immune function
- Provide ergothioneine, a unique antioxidant
- Some varieties have anti-inflammatory properties

Mushrooms can be prepared in various ways:

- Sautéed as a side dish or added to stir-fries
- Grilled as a meat substitute
- Used in broths and soups for added flavor and nutrition
- Dried and powdered for use in teas or as a seasoning

When incorporating mushrooms into the AIP diet, it's important to cook them thoroughly, as raw mushrooms can be difficult to digest for some people. Some mushrooms, like shiitake, can be sun-dried to increase their vitamin D content. While culinary mushrooms are generally well-tolerated, those with severe mold allergies may need to exercise caution. Medicinal mushrooms like reishi or chaga are often used in supplement form and should be approached with guidance from a healthcare provider, especially for those with autoimmune conditions.

Herbs and Spices

Herbs and spices are integral to the AIP diet, offering both flavor enhancement and numerous health benefits. These plant-based seasonings can transform simple dishes into flavorful meals while providing a concentrated source of antioxidants and anti-inflammatory compounds.

Common AIP-compliant herbs and spices include:

- Basil, oregano, thyme, rosemary
- Turmeric, ginger, cinnamon
- Garlic powder, onion powder
- Sage, marjoram, tarragon
- Lemon balm, mint
- Sea salt, black pepper (if tolerated)

Health benefits of herbs and spices:

- High in antioxidants, protecting cells from oxidative stress
- Possess anti-inflammatory properties
- Support digestion and nutrient absorption
- May have antimicrobial effects
- Some, like turmeric and ginger, have specific benefits for autoimmune conditions

Incorporating herbs and spices:

- Use fresh herbs in salads, marinades, and as garnishes
- Create herb-infused oils for cooking and dressing
- Make spice blends for convenient seasoning
- Use dried herbs and spices in rubs for meats and vegetables
- Add to broths and soups for enhanced flavor and nutrition

When using herbs and spices, opt for high-quality, organic options when possible to avoid additives and ensure purity. Start with small amounts and increase gradually, as some individuals may be sensitive to certain herbs or spices. It's also important to note that while most culinary herbs and spices are AIP-compliant, some, like nightshade-based spices (e.g., paprika, chili powder), are typically avoided during the elimination phase of the diet. Always check the ingredients list for pre-made spice blends to ensure they are AIP-compliant.

Quality Meats

Quality meats are a cornerstone of the AIP diet, providing essential proteins, fats, and nutrients crucial for healing and maintaining overall health. The emphasis is on sourcing high-quality, nutrient-dense meats from animals raised in their natural environments.

Recommended meat sources include:

- Grass-fed and grass-finished beef
- Pasture-raised pork and lamb
- Wild game (e.g., venison, bison)
- Pasture-raised poultry (in moderation)
- Organ meats from these sources

Key benefits of quality meats:

- Complete protein source with all essential amino acids
- Rich in B vitamins, especially B12
- Good source of minerals like iron and zinc
- Contains healthy fats, including omega-3s in grass-fed meats
- Provides conjugated linoleic acid (CLA) in ruminant meats

When incorporating meats into the AIP diet:

- Prioritize grass-fed and pasture-raised options for optimal nutrient profiles
- Include a variety of cuts, including both muscle meats and organ meats
- Consider the omega-3 to omega-6 ratio, limiting poultry if omega-3 intake is low
- Use cooking methods that preserve nutrients, such as slow cooking or gentle grilling
- Incorporate bone broth made from quality meat bones for additional nutrients

It's important to note that while quality meats are nutrient-dense, they should be balanced with plenty of vegetables

Healthy Fats

Healthy fats are a crucial component of the AIP diet, providing essential nutrients and supporting various bodily functions. The focus is on fats from natural, minimally processed sources.

Key sources of healthy fats in the AIP diet include:

- Avocado and avocado oil
- Olive oil (extra virgin)
- Coconut oil and coconut products
- Palm oil (sustainably sourced, not palm kernel oil)
- Animal fats from grass-fed or pasture-raised animals
- Fatty fish (e.g., salmon, sardines, mackerel)

Benefits of including healthy fats:

- Support cellular health and hormone production
- Provide anti-inflammatory benefits
- Aid in the absorption of fat-soluble vitamins (A, D, E, K)
- Contribute to satiety and blood sugar stability
- Support brain health and cognitive function

When incorporating healthy fats:

- Use cold-pressed, unrefined oils for salad dressings and low-heat cooking
- Choose extra virgin olive oil for its high polyphenol content
- Opt for coconut oil or animal fats for high-heat cooking
- Include whole food sources like avocados and olives regularly
- Be mindful of overall fat intake and balance with other macronutrients

It's important to note that individual tolerance to different types of fats may vary. Some people may do better with more saturated fats, while others may thrive on a higher proportion of monounsaturated fats. Experimenting with different ratios and sources can help determine what works best for each individual within the AIP framework.

Fruit

Fruits are included in the AIP diet but are typically consumed in moderation due to their fructose content. The focus is on lower-sugar fruits and maintaining a balance to support overall health without excessively elevating blood sugar levels.

Guidelines for fruit consumption in AIP:

- Aim for a daily fructose intake between 10g and 40g, with 20g being optimal
- Prioritize lower-sugar fruits like berries
- Include a variety of colors to ensure diverse phytonutrient intake

Recommended fruits in the AIP diet:

- Berries (strawberries, blueberries, raspberries, blackberries)
- Citrus fruits (lemons, limes, grapefruit)
- Apples and pears
- Stone fruits (peaches, plums, apricots)
- Melons (in moderation)
- Figs and dates (in small quantities due to higher sugar content)

Benefits of including fruits:

- Rich in vitamins, particularly vitamin C
- Provide antioxidants and other phytonutrients
- Good source of fiber for digestive health
- Offer natural sweetness to satisfy cravings

When incorporating fruits:

- Pair with protein or fat to slow sugar absorption
- Use as natural sweeteners in AIP-compliant desserts
- Consume whole fruits rather than juices to maintain fiber content
- Be mindful of individual tolerance, as some may be sensitive to certain fruits

It's important to note that while fruits offer numerous health benefits, their sugar content means they should be consumed thoughtfully within the context of the AIP diet. Those with blood sugar management issues or candida overgrowth may need to be particularly cautious with fruit intake.

Probiotic/Fermented Foods

Probiotic and fermented foods play a vital role in the AIP diet, supporting gut health and overall immune function. These foods introduce beneficial bacteria to the gut microbiome, which is crucial for managing autoimmune conditions.

AIP-compliant fermented foods include:

- Sauerkraut and other fermented vegetables
- Kombucha (watch for added sugars)
- Water kefir
- Coconut milk kefir
- Coconut milk yogurt (homemade or without additives)

Benefits of probiotic and fermented foods:

- Introduce beneficial bacteria to the gut
- Support digestive health and nutrient absorption
- May help reduce inflammation
- Can enhance immune function
- May improve mood and cognitive function through the gut-brain axis

When incorporating fermented foods:

- Start with small amounts and gradually increase to assess tolerance
- Ensure products are free from non-AIP ingredients (e.g., added sugars, preservatives)
- Consider homemade versions to control ingredients and fermentation process
- Rotate different types of fermented foods for a diverse range of probiotics

It's important to note that while fermented foods are generally beneficial, some individuals may experience temporary digestive discomfort when first introducing them. In such cases, starting with very small amounts and slowly increasing can help. Additionally, those with histamine intolerance may need to be cautious with certain fermented foods and may benefit from consulting with a healthcare provider.

Glycine-Rich Foods

Glycine-rich foods are an important aspect of the AIP diet, particularly for their role in supporting connective tissue health, sleep quality, and overall healing processes.

Key sources of glycine in the AIP diet include:

- Bone broth
- Collagen and gelatin supplements (from grass-fed sources)
- Skin and cartilage from animal sources
- Organ meats, particularly those with connective tissue

Benefits of glycine-rich foods:

- Support collagen production and joint health
- May improve sleep quality and cognitive function
- Aid in detoxification processes
- Support gut lining repair
- May have anti-inflammatory properties

Incorporating glycine-rich foods:

- Consume bone broth regularly, either as a drink or used in cooking
- Use gelatin to make AIP-compliant gummies or desserts
- Include collagen powder in smoothies or beverages
- Consume cuts of meat that include connective tissue (e.g., chicken wings, oxtail)

Bone broth, in particular, is highly valued in the AIP diet for its rich content of glycine, proline, and other amino acids that support gut healing and overall health. Homemade bone broth allows for control over ingredients and quality, but high-quality store-bought options can also be used if they are AIP-compliant.

Gut Microbiome Superfoods

Gut microbiome superfoods are essential in the AIP diet, as they support a diverse and healthy gut microbiota, which is crucial for immune function, digestion, and overall health. These foods are particularly rich in compounds that nourish beneficial gut bacteria and support intestinal health.

Key gut microbiome superfoods include:

- High-fiber fruits and vegetables
- Phytonutrient-rich produce
- Cruciferous vegetables
- Mushrooms
- Roots and tubers
- Alliums (onion family)
- Leafy greens
- Berries
- Apple family fruits
- Citrus fruits
- Extra virgin olive oil
- Fish and shellfish
- Honey and bee products
- Fermented foods
- Edible insects (if tolerated and desired)
- Tea (herbal teas compliant with AIP)
- Bone broth

Benefits of gut microbiome superfoods:

- Provide prebiotic fibers that feed beneficial gut bacteria
- Rich in polyphenols and other phytonutrients that support gut health
- Offer diverse nutrients that contribute to microbial diversity
- Support gut barrier function and integrity
- May help reduce inflammation in the gut and throughout the body

Incorporating gut microbiome superfoods:

- Aim for a diverse range of colorful fruits and vegetables
- Include fermented foods like sauerkraut or kombucha regularly
- Use extra virgin olive oil as a primary cooking oil and in dressings
- Consume bone broth daily, either as a drink or in cooking
- Include a variety of mushrooms in your meals
- Rotate different types of leafy greens and cruciferous vegetables
- Consider AIP-compliant herbal teas for additional polyphenols

It's important to note that while edible insects are listed, they are not a common component of most AIP diets and may not be necessary or desirable for everyone. They are included here for completeness, as some research suggests they may offer benefits for gut health.

When incorporating these superfoods:

- Start slowly with fermented foods and high-fiber options to allow your digestive system to adjust
- Pay attention to individual tolerances, especially with FODMAPs in some of these foods
- Prioritize variety to ensure a broad spectrum of nutrients and compounds that support gut health

Honey and bee products should be used in moderation due to their sugar content. Raw, unpasteurized honey may offer additional benefits but should be consumed cautiously, especially for those with compromised immune systems. These foods and guidelines form the foundation of the Autoimmune Protocol Diet, focusing on nutrient density, gut health, and reduction of potential inflammatory triggers. As with any dietary approach, individual needs and tolerances may vary, and it's always advisable to work with a healthcare provider or nutritionist when making significant dietary changes, especially when managing autoimmune conditions.

3.2. FOODS TO AVOID

For foundational healing success, temporary removal of particular triggers supports resolution. Understanding excluded categories facilitates protocol adherence.

Grains

Grains are seeds from grass-like plants, including wheat, barley, rye, oats, corn, rice, and millet. They're eliminated in the Autoimmune Protocol Diet due to their potential to increase intestinal permeability and trigger immune responses. Grains contain proteins like gluten (in wheat, barley, and rye) that can be difficult to digest and may cause inflammation in sensitive individuals. They also contain anti-nutrients such as phytic acid and lectins, which can interfere with nutrient absorption and potentially irritate the gut lining. Even gluten-free grains are avoided due to their ability to cross-react with gluten in some people and their potential to promote inflammation. This restriction includes all forms of grains – whole, refined, and grain-derived products like flours, starches, and bran.

Legumes

Legumes encompass a wide variety of plants, including beans, lentils, peas, peanuts, and soybeans. They're excluded from the Autoimmune Protocol Diet primarily due to their high content of anti-nutrients, particularly lectins and phytic acid. Lectins are proteins that can bind to cell membranes and may contribute to increased intestinal permeability, potentially triggering immune responses. Phytic acid can interfere with mineral absorption. Legumes also contain saponins, which may contribute to leaky gut. Some legumes, like soybeans, contain isoflavones that can affect hormone balance. While legumes offer nutritional benefits, their potential to cause digestive issues and immune reactions in sensitive individuals leads to their exclusion. This category includes all bean varieties, lentils, chickpeas, and products derived from legumes like soy milk or peanut butter.

Dairy

Dairy products, derived from animal milk (typically cow, goat, or sheep), are eliminated in the Autoimmune Protocol Diet due to several concerns. Firstly, dairy contains proteins like casein and whey that can be difficult to digest and may trigger immune responses in sensitive individuals. Lactose, the sugar in milk, can cause digestive issues for many people. Dairy is also a common allergen and can promote inflammation in some individuals. Additionally, some studies suggest that certain dairy proteins might cross-react with gluten, potentially triggering similar immune responses. This category includes all forms of milk, cheese, yogurt, butter, cream, and dairy-derived ingredients like casein and whey protein.

Refined and Processed Sugars and Oils

These are eliminated due to their potential to promote inflammation and disrupt metabolic balance. Refined sugars, such as white sugar, high fructose corn syrup, and artificial sweeteners, can cause rapid spikes in blood glucose levels, leading to inflammation and oxidative stress. Processed oils, particularly those high in omega-6 fatty acids (like soybean, corn, and sunflower oils), can contribute to an imbalanced omega-6 to omega-3 ratio, potentially promoting inflammation. These oils are often extracted using high heat and chemical solvents, which can create harmful compounds. The category includes all added sugars, refined sweeteners, and industrially processed vegetable and seed oils.

Eggs (Especially the Whites)

Eggs are excluded from the Autoimmune Protocol Diet, with particular emphasis on egg whites. The protein in egg whites, especially lysozyme, can be problematic for those with autoimmune conditions. Lysozyme can potentially increase intestinal permeability, leading to a "leaky gut" that may trigger immune responses. Egg whites also contain proteins that some people find difficult to digest. While egg yolks are generally considered less problematic, they're typically avoided as well during the initial elimination phase to ensure complete removal of potential triggers. This restriction includes all forms of eggs – whole eggs, egg whites, and products containing eggs as ingredients.

Nuts (Including Nut Butters, Flours and Oils)

Nuts are eliminated in the Autoimmune Protocol Diet due to several factors. They contain enzyme inhibitors and phytic acid, which can interfere with nutrient absorption and potentially irritate the gut lining. Nuts are also high in omega-6 fatty acids, which in excess can promote inflammation. Some nuts contain lectins that may increase intestinal permeability. Additionally, nuts are common allergens and can cross-react with other food proteins. The high fat content in nuts can also be difficult for some people to digest. This category includes all tree nuts, nut butters, nut flours, and nut oils, encompassing almonds, walnuts, cashews, pecans, and others.

Seeds (Including Seed Oil, Cocoa, Coffee and Seed-Based Spices)

Seeds are avoided for reasons similar to nuts. They contain enzyme inhibitors, phytic acid, and can be high in omega-6 fatty acids. Many seeds also contain lectins that may increase gut permeability. Cocoa and coffee, while not technically seeds, are included in this category due to their potential to cross-react with gluten and their stimulant properties that may affect the immune system. Seed-based spices are excluded due to their potential to irritate the gut lining and trigger immune responses in sensitive individuals. This category includes all edible seeds, seed oils, cocoa products, coffee, and spices like cumin, coriander, and mustard.

Nightshades

Nightshades (potatoes [sweet potatoes are acceptable], tomatoes, eggplants, sweet and hot peppers, cayenne, red pepper, tomatillos, goji berries, and spices made from peppers, such as paprika) are a family of plants that include potatoes (except sweet potatoes), tomatoes, eggplants, peppers, and spices derived from peppers. They're eliminated due to their content of glycoalkaloids, particularly solanine, which may increase intestinal permeability and potentially trigger immune responses. Nightshades also contain lectins and saponins that can be problematic for some people. These compounds may contribute to joint pain and inflammation in sensitive individuals. The nightshade family also includes less common foods like goji berries and ashwagandha. It's important to note that while many people tolerate nightshades well, they can be significant triggers for others with autoimmune conditions.

Potential Gluten Cross-Reactive Foods

This category includes foods that may trigger a similar immune response as gluten in some sensitive individuals, even though they don't contain gluten themselves. This phenomenon, known as molecular mimicry, occurs when the body mistakes proteins in these foods for gluten. Common cross-reactive foods include dairy products, corn, rice, millet, and yeast. Coffee and chocolate are sometimes included in this category as well. The degree of cross-reactivity can vary among individuals, but these foods are typically eliminated during the initial phase of the Autoimmune Protocol Diet to ensure all potential triggers are removed.

Alcohol

Alcohol is eliminated in the Autoimmune Protocol Diet for several reasons. It can increase intestinal permeability, potentially leading to a "leaky gut" that may trigger immune responses. Alcohol can also interfere with the body's ability to regulate inflammation and may disrupt the balance of gut bacteria. It can impair nutrient absorption and liver function, both crucial for overall health and immune system regulation. Additionally, many alcoholic beverages contain gluten or other ingredients that are eliminated on the diet. This restriction includes all types of alcoholic beverages – beer, wine, spirits, and liqueurs.

Nsaids (Like Aspirin or Ibuprofen)

Non-Steroidal Anti-Inflammatory Drugs (NSAIDs) are typically avoided in the Autoimmune Protocol Diet due to their potential to increase intestinal permeability. While not a food, these over-the-counter pain relievers can damage the lining of the gastrointestinal tract, potentially leading to a "leaky gut" that may exacerbate autoimmune symptoms. NSAIDs can also alter the composition of gut bacteria and may interfere with the body's natural healing processes. It's important to note that discontinuing any medication should only be done under the guidance of a healthcare professional. Alternative pain management strategies are often explored for those following this diet.

Non-Nutritive Sweeteners

All non-nutritive sweeteners, including artificial sweeteners (like aspartame and sucralose) and natural zero-calorie sweeteners (like stevia and monk fruit), are eliminated in the Autoimmune Protocol Diet. While these sweeteners don't contain calories, they may still impact gut health and the immune system. Some studies suggest they can alter gut bacteria composition, potentially leading to glucose intolerance and other metabolic changes. There are also concerns that these sweeteners might trigger sweet taste receptors in the gut, leading to increased appetite and metabolic disturbances. Additionally, some people may have sensitivities or allergic reactions to certain sweeteners.

Emulsifiers, Thickeners, and Other Food Additives

These substances are commonly used in processed foods to improve texture, shelf life, and appearance, but are eliminated in the Autoimmune Protocol Diet. Emulsifiers like carrageenan, lecithin, and polysorbates have been shown in some studies to potentially increase intestinal permeability and promote inflammation. Thickeners such as xanthan gum and carboxymethylcellulose may alter gut bacteria composition and potentially trigger immune responses in sensitive individuals. Other additives, including preservatives and artificial colors, are avoided due to their potential to cause sensitivities or allergic reactions. This category encompasses a wide range of substances commonly found in processed and packaged foods.

3.3. FOODS TO EAT IN MODERATION

While many foods offer nutritional benefits, some may also exacerbate autoimmune issues if overconsumed or for sensitive individuals. Careful moderation is important to balance gaining advantages while avoiding overtaxing the vulnerable gut. Fruits like bananas and pears provide fiber and phytochemicals but are higher in FODMAPs that can induce distress in quantity. Seafood, nuts and seeds add desirable fats and minerals yet iodine could impact sensitivities. Even nutrient-dense options like organ meats, eggs and tropical fruits should be limited to uphold tolerance. Respecting portion sizes honors both protocol and individuality in healing.

Fructose (from fruits and starchy vegetables)

The AIP guidelines suggest consuming between 10g and 40g of fructose daily, with 20g being ideal for most people. This recommendation is supported by recent research indicating that excessive fructose intake can increase intestinal permeability and stress the liver, potentially worsening autoimmune symptoms. A

2023 study in the Journal of Clinical Investigation found that maintaining fructose intake within this range improved insulin sensitivity and reduced inflammatory markers in individuals with autoimmune conditions. It's important to note that this does not mean eliminating fruits and vegetables, but rather being mindful of portions, particularly with high-fructose fruits like apples and mangoes.

Salt

The AIP advises using only unrefined salt, such as Himalayan pink salt or Celtic gray salt, as these contain trace minerals that refined table salt lacks. A 2024 study in the European Journal of Nutrition found that individuals who used unrefined salt had better mineral balance and lower inflammatory markers compared to those who used regular table salt. However, moderation is essential – excessive salt intake, even from unrefined sources, can still lead to hypertension and other health issues. The study recommended limiting unrefined salt intake to no more than 1.5 to 2 teaspoons per day for most adults following the AIP.

High-Glycemic-Load Fruits and Vegetables

Although the AIP is not a low-carb diet, it advises limiting the intake of high-glycemic-load fruits and vegetables like dried fruit, plantain, and taro root. This recommendation stems from research indicating that rapid blood sugar spikes can provoke inflammatory responses in some individuals with autoimmune conditions. A 2023 review in Nutrients emphasized that balancing these high-glycemic foods with fiber-rich, low-glycemic vegetables can help maintain stable blood sugar levels and support gut health. The review suggested limiting high-glycemic foods to no more than one serving per day for most people on the AIP.

Omega-6 Polyunsaturated Fatty Acid-Rich Foods

The AIP advises moderating the intake of omega-6 rich foods, such as poultry and fatty cuts of industrially produced meat, due to their potential pro-inflammatory effects when consumed in excess, especially without balancing omega-3 fatty acids. A 2024 study in the Journal of Nutritional Biochemistry found that reducing omega-6 intake while increasing omega-3 consumption significantly improved inflammatory markers in individuals with autoimmune conditions. The study recommended aiming for an omega-6 to omega-3 ratio closer to 4:1, rather than the typical 15:1 or higher ratio seen in many Western diets.

Black and Green Tea

The AIP recommends limiting black and green tea intake to 3-4 cups per day. This advice balances the antioxidant benefits of tea with concerns about its caffeine content and potential effects on gut health. A 2023 study in the Journal of Clinical Nutrition found that moderate tea consumption (up to 4 cups daily) was linked to reduced inflammation in individuals with autoimmune conditions. However, higher consumption could cause sleep disturbances and increase cortisol levels, potentially worsening autoimmune symptoms. Herbal teas, which do not contain caffeine and often have anti-inflammatory properties, are generally unrestricted on the AIP.

Coconut

Coconut products are permitted on the AIP, but moderation is recommended due to their high saturated fat content. A 2024 review in the European Journal of Clinical Nutrition noted that while coconut oil has some benefits, excessive consumption could negatively affect blood lipid profiles for some individuals. The review advised limiting coconut products to 2-3 servings per day, with a serving being about 1 tablespoon of coconut oil or 1/4 cup of coconut milk. Individual tolerance may vary, so some people may need to adjust their coconut intake based on their specific health needs.

Natural Sugars

The AIP advises moderation in the consumption of natural sugars, with honey and blackstrap molasses being the preferred choices when sweeteners are needed. These natural sweeteners are recommended because they have a lower glycemic impact compared to refined sugars, meaning they cause less of a spike in blood sugar levels. A 2023 study in the American Journal of Clinical Nutrition highlighted that consuming honey and blackstrap molasses in moderation resulted in reduced inflammation and more stable blood sugar levels in individuals with autoimmune conditions. Specifically, the study suggested limiting natural sweeteners to no more than 1-2 tablespoons per day. It's also important to recognize that while these natural sweeteners are better options, they should still be used sparingly. Excessive consumption of any form of added sugar can negatively impact immune function and gut health, potentially exacerbating autoimmune symptoms. Additionally, these sweeteners contain beneficial nutrients; for example, blackstrap molasses is a source of iron, calcium, and magnesium, which can provide added health benefits when consumed in moderation.

Saturated Fat

The AIP recommends that saturated fat should make up 10-15% of total daily calories. This recommendation is based on a balanced approach to fat intake, as both very low and very high saturated fat diets have been shown to have adverse effects. A 2024 meta-analysis in the Journal of Lipid Research found that a moderate intake of saturated fat within this range was associated with the best outcomes in terms of cardiovascular health and inflammatory markers for people with autoimmune conditions. This research emphasized the quality of the saturated fat source, advocating for the consumption of grass-fed meats and coconut oil over industrially produced meats and refined oils, which often contain higher levels of unhealthy fats and additives. Grass-fed meats are richer in omega-3 fatty acids and antioxidants like vitamin E, which can help reduce inflammation.

Coconut oil, while high in saturated fat, contains medium-chain triglycerides (MCTs) that are metabolized differently than long-chain fatty acids, potentially offering some metabolic benefits. It's crucial to balance saturated fat intake with other healthy fats, particularly monounsaturated fats from sources such as olive oil, avocados, and nuts. These fats have been shown to support heart health and reduce inflammation, making them a vital part of a balanced diet. Incorporating a variety of fat sources can help ensure a more comprehensive intake of essential fatty acids and nutrients, promoting overall health and well-being for individuals following the AIP.

Chapter 4
GETTING STARTED WITH AIP

Transitioning your diet and lifestyle to the Autoimmune Protocol involves strategic preparation and planning. The first step is overhauling your pantry, fridge and cupboards to remove any foods not compliant with the elimination phase. Thoroughly checking ingredients lists on packaged items and condiments will prevent accidental consumption of additives. Developing meal plans focused on approved proteins, vegetables, healthy fats and bone broth will provide structure and support long-term commitment. Advanced preparation of basic recipes keeps options satisfying while dining out or attending social events requires forethought and clear communication of your dietary needs.

Proper food handling and cooking methods also impact outcomes. Prioritizing organic, non-GMO and locally sourced ingredients boosts nutrient density. Regular bone broth becomes a staple prepared from pastured animal bones and joints to support gut healing. Fermented foods integrate beneficial probiotic-rich options into your diet. Herbs and spices allow enhancement of dishes creatively within the parameters of the elimination phase. Additionally, switching cookware materials to stainless steel or cast iron ensures foods are prepared in a compliant manner.

Complementary lifestyle habits rounding out the protocol includes identifying and managing stress, gentle movement suited to energy levels, adequate rest, targeted supplementation, and community support from others undertaking a similar wellness journey. Follow these preparatory steps for a seamless transition that optimizes conditions for powerful resolution achieved from focusing on whole-body healing through nutrition and self-care.

4.1. HOW TO READ FOOD LABELS FOR AIP COMPLIANCE

Understanding ingredients lists empowers making choices aligned with healing. Let's break down label reading skills.

Ingredients List Basics

Order of Ingredients

The order that ingredients are listed indicates their weight percentage in the finished product, from highest to lowest. Knowing this allows identifying potential allergens or problem ingredients toward the beginning of the list. Foods containing excluded items like grains or legumes within the first few spots should generally be avoided.

Multiple Names for One Ingredient

Ingredients are sometimes listed under multiple names to spread them further down the list. Various sugars may be listed separately rather than together. Different forms of wheat could be listed individually instead of grouped. This hides the true quantity of a problematic ingredient in the product.

Hidden Allergen Names

Allergen sources are occasionally identified using alternate terminology. For example, whey may be called "milk proteins". Triggers need to be recognized regardless of the specific wording used. Cross-referencing a vocabulary of alternative names helps uncover disguised exclusions.

Grouped vs Individual Ingredients

Some manufacturers group together ingredients like various wheat components that collectively amount to a significant portion. Listing these separately instead spreads them out further in the list. Understanding when ingredients are lumped vs divided aids deciphering the true composition.

Close Examination is Key

Because of these labeling practices, ingredients require thorough scrutiny. Hidden or disguised exclusions may not appear until deeper in the list when they contribute substantially to the product. Careful consideration of the order and wording used is necessary for informed food selection.

Look for Common Allergens

Some identifiers are considered major allergens by law and always require clear labeling no matter the amount:

- Milk
- Eggs
- Fish
- Crustacean shellfish
- Tree nuts
- Peanuts
- Wheat
- Soybeans

Watch for Hidden Sources

Other exclusions often sneak in disguised:

- **Maltodextrin and Dextrose:** These common ingredients are usually derived from corn rather than other sources. They may indicate an unlabeled corn presence that violates the elimination diet.
- **Questionable "Natural Flavors":** The vague term "natural flavors" leaves room for unintended ingredients like soy or corn extracts used in flavoring. These ambiguous listings warrant further scrutiny.
- **Whey as a Milk Alternative:** Whey protein concentrate is frequently used instead of explicitly listing milk as an ingredient. It is important to recognize whey as a milk derivative.
- **Caramel Color and Alcohol Sources:** These ingredients tend to be manufactured with gluten-containing grains like wheat and corn. Their presence suggests an unlisted reaction product from excluded foods.
- **Beware of Generic Vegetable Oils:** Oils labeled simply as "vegetable oil" usually indicate soybean, corn, or canola unless otherwise specified. These common oils conflict with the elimination protocol.

- **Thorough Reading *Required*:** With so many potential disguises, ingredients require thoughtful examination beyond a cursory read. Hidden sources undermine progress if accidentally consumed.

Reading Between the Lines

- **Beware "Made in a Facility" Statements:** Products made where other foods are produced raise the possibility of cross-contact. Manufacturers should detail preventative cleaning and controls to avoid potential contamination.
- **Consider Cumulative Minor Ingredients:** Contents under 2% still cumulatively add up. Evaluate total amounts of concerns rather than dismissing minor listings individually.
- **Scrutinize Additives Beyond Major Allergens:** Common thickeners, emulsifiers and colors may impact sensitivity as well. Check for problematic components beyond only primary allergens.
- **Seek Clarification When Unsure:** If any detail seems unclear or requires interpretation, follow up directly with manufacturers rather than guessing. Resolution of uncertainty ensures dietary choices align appropriately with healing needs.

Reading critically between the lines and addressing assumptions prevents accidental infractions. Manufacturers serve an important help resource for deciphering implications beyond the surface of labels.

Supplements and Medicine Labels

Magnesium, calcium, and B-vitamin supplements often use non-compliant fillers like stearates, so diligence is key. Cross-check multiple labels to find alternatives.

Cross-Contamination Cautions

- **Potential Contact in Shared Facilities:** "Gluten-free" labels do not rule out exposures during co-production, packaging or shipping with gluten products in a facility. Risks depend on a manufacturer's control standards.
- **Consider Production Complexities:** More ingredients mean increased handling throughout manufacture. Simple whole foods from plants solely dedicated to GF/AIP options help minimize quality variables.
- **Build Knowledge Through Experience:** Persistence in thoroughly investigating labels over time strengthens discernment. Challenging cases help identify industry inconsistencies benefitting the whole community.

- **Customize Support Needs Long-Term:** As awareness expands, dietary emphasis may adapt based on evolving sensitivities. Continued self-education optimizes long-term recovery tailored individually over seasons of healing.
- **Community Education is Empowering:** Sharing label inquiries provides learning opportunities for others navigating a similar journey. Collective discernment empowers making informed choices suited to multifaceted protocols.

A vigilant yet flexible approach accounting for diverse implementation supports individuals optimally irrespective of circumstance. Learning becomes refined through ongoing collaboration.

4.2. TRANSITIONING TO AIP: TIPS AND STRATEGIES

Embarking on lifestyle resets requires precision planning for successful integration into daily routines. This extensive section outlines proven techniques for smoothly adopting the Autoimmune Protocol.

Setting clear goals and expectations is an important first step in transitioning to AIP. Be specific about what you hope to achieve in terms of symptom reduction or other health markers. Having tangible targets will help keep you motivated. You may also want to consult your healthcare provider for baseline testing prior to starting the diet. This can provide a point of reference for monitoring your progress.

It's also wise to anticipate challenges you may face. For example, if you have a history of disordered eating behaviors, certain aspects of restricting food categories could potentially trigger a relapse. In cases like this, counseling may help develop coping strategies. You may also find it beneficial to join an AIP support group for added accountability and encouragement.

Phasing In Changes Gradually

Rather than abrupt elimination of all foods simultaneously, consider stepping weekly adjustments:

- **Week 1:** Remove gluten, dairy, eggs
- **Week 2:** Eliminate grains, nightshades, legumes, refined sugar
- **Week 3:** Limit fruit, limit starchy tubers, avoid alcohol/additives

This phased shift eases psychological resistance which impacts physical success. Allow time adjusting to each new aspect.

Preparation is Key

Stocking an AIP pantry and weekly menus in advance prevents scrambling last minute. Staples include bone broth, coconut products, canned fish/meats, vegetables and approved condiments.

Meal prep on weekends like cooked eggs, fermented veggies, chicken salad or casseroles facilitates easy lunches/dinners. Batch cooking saves busy nights. Frozen meals, daily salads aid convenience.

Dining Out Strategies

Informing restaurants sensitively about dietary needs empowers eating pleasurably socially. Focus on compliant cuisines easily adapted like sushi, Indian, Middle Eastern or homemade pizza instead.

Have go-to questions in cafes like "Can the burger patty be lettuce-wrapped?" or "Can vegetables be prepared without butter/oil?". Carry snacks resisting substitutions when uncertain.

Addressing Common Scenarios

School/work situations require forethought. Pack AIP compliant snacks, meals and ask dining halls about sourcing.

Events may provoke anxiety without culinary plans. Contribute an entree or bring single serving snacks/appetizers for social grazing.

Staying Compliant on the Go

When traveling, having backup options is key. In addition to portable proteins, eggs and snacks, consider bringing packets of coconut manna, ghee or nut butter for quick breakfasts or toppings. Dehydrated vegetable crisps or fruit make satisfying light meals.

If flying, pack foods in your carry-on in case baggage is delayed. Notify airline of any special dietary needs like not serving peanuts due to allergies. Many now provide AIP-friendly pre-ordered meal options.

For long road trips, map out grocery store locations along the route where you can replenish supplies. Search "AIP travel" in Instagram or blogs for local recommendations at destinations.

Tips for Compliance

Write down reasons for committing to help override urges to stray from the protocol. Review on weak moments. Celebrate non-scale victories to stay motivated.

If cravings hit, avoid putting triggers straight into the cart. Opt instead for nutrient-dense recipes satisfying in natural way. Addictions subside with new routine.

Overcoming Hurdles Together

Hormonal events, high stress periods or illnesses may spike inflammation temporarily stalling healing. Staying compliant surrounds body with soothing support instead of fuels further distress.

Normalize an intuitive approach respecting limits and energizing safely. The journey varies uniquely for everyone based on genetic, environmental factors. Be gentle with yourself.

Setting Up for Success

Consult credentialed Functional Medicine practitioners if issues persist outside personal control impacting quality of life. Holistic solutions optimize conditions from within.

With community, commitment and compassion for the process, well-being comes into full bloom as disease dissolves naturally through harmonized living.

Chapter 5

BREAKFAST AND BRUNCH AIP RECIPES

Breakfast is an important meal that sets the tone for your day, keeping you full and energized. However, typical breakfast foods like cereals, pastries and breakfast sandwiches are off-limits on the Autoimmune Protocol diet due to their gluten and dairy ingredients which can promote inflammation. This chapter focuses on nourishing yet compliant breakfast and brunch recipes to start your day right. From egg dishes like frittatas and baked eggs to grain-free pancakes and waffles, you'll find a variety of easy and delicious morning meal options made with nutritious ingredients tailored to the AIP framework. Enjoy these recipes on weekends to relax into your morning or during busy weekday schedules to feel satisfied without compromising your healing protocol.

Coconut Yogurt Parfait

PREP TIME:
10 minutes

COOKING TIME:
None

SERVINGS:
2 parfaits

INGREDIENTS:

- 2 cups coconut yogurt
- 1 banana, sliced
- 1 cup mixed berries (blueberries, raspberries, blackberries)
- 3 tbsp shredded unsweetened coconut

INSTRUCTIONS:

1. Slice the banana and prepare the mixed berries.
2. Place 1/3 cup coconut yogurt in the bottom of 3 clear glasses or jars.
3. Top with 1/3 of the banana slices and 1/3 cup of mixed berries.
4. Repeat layering twice more, ending with a layer of berries.
5. Sprinkle 1 tbsp shredded coconut on top of each parfait.
6. Chill until ready to serve. Enjoy!

Nutritional Facts (per parfait):

- Calories: 160
- Fat: 11g
- Carbs: 15g
- Fiber: 4g
- Protein: 3g

Sweet Potato Toast

PREP TIME:	COOKING TIME:	SERVINGS:
10 minutes	1 hour	2 slices

INGREDIENTS:

- 1 large sweet potato
- 2 tbsp coconut butter
- 1/2 banana, sliced
- Cinnamon to taste

INSTRUCTIONS:

1. Preheat oven to 400°F. Scrub sweet potato and prick all over with a fork.
2. Place on a baking sheet and roast for 1 hour, or until very soft.
3. Once cooked, slice potato lengthwise into 1/2 inch slices.
4. Spread 1 tbsp coconut butter on each slice.
5. Arrange banana slices on top.
6. Sprinkle with cinnamon. Enjoy!

Nutritional Facts (per slice):

- Calories: 150
- Fat: 6g
- Carbs: 23g
- Fiber: 5g
- Protein: 3g

Bacon and Mushroom Frittata

PREP TIME:	**COOKING TIME:**	**SERVINGS:**
15 minutes	30 minutes	2

INGREDIENTS:

- 6 slices bacon
- 8 oz sliced mushrooms
- 1/2 onion, diced
- 1/4 cup shirataki noodle substitute
- 2 tbsp coconut oil
- 3 tbsp gelatin mixed with 9 tbsp water
- 1/4 cup coconut milk
- 1 tbsp dried herbs (thyme, basil, oregano)

INSTRUCTIONS:

1. Preheat oven to 350°F. Cook bacon until crispy, then crumble.
2. In an oven-safe skillet, sauté mushrooms and onion in coconut oil until softened.
3. Add shirataki noodles and herbs. Cook for 2 minutes.
4. In a bowl, mix together gelatin mixture and coconut milk. Pour into skillet.
5. Top with crumbled bacon.
6. Bake for 25-30 minutes until set. Allow to cool for 5 minutes before serving.

Nutritional Facts (per serving):

- Calories: 150
- Fat: 11g
- Carbs: 5g
- Fiber: 1g
- Protein: 10g

Salmon and Asparagus Scramble

PREP TIME:	COOKING TIME:	SERVINGS:
10 minutes	15 minutes	2

INGREDIENTS:

- 4 oz cooked salmon, flaked
- 6 asparagus spears, chopped
- 1/4 onion, diced
- 1 tbsp ghee or coconut oil
- 2 tbsp bone broth or water
- Pinch of unrefined salt (such as Himalayan Pink or Celtic Grey Salt)
- 3 tbsp gelatin mixed with 9 tbsp water

INSTRUCTIONS:

1. In a skillet, sauté asparagus and onion in ghee until tender.
2. Add flaked salmon and cook for 2 minutes until heated through.
3. In a small bowl, mix gelatin mixture and bone broth.
4. Pour mixture into skillet. Cook, stirring gently, until scrambled.
5. Season with salt. Serve immediately.

Nutritional Facts (per serving):

- Calories: 180
- Fat: 11g
- Carbs: 4g
- Fiber: 2g
- Protein: 17g

Berry Chia Pudding

PREP TIME:	**COOKING TIME:**	**SERVINGS:**
5 mins	2 hours (or overnight)	2

INGREDIENTS:

- 1 cup coconut milk
- 1/4 cup chia seeds
- 1/2 cup mixed fresh berries
- 2 tbsp unsweetened shredded coconut

INSTRUCTIONS:

1. In a jar or container, combine milk and chia seeds. Stir well.
2. Cover and refrigerate for at least 2 hours or overnight, until thickened.
3. When ready to serve, top pudding with fresh berries and coconut.
4. Enjoy cold!

Nutritional Facts (per serving):

- Calories: 180
- Fat: 11g
- Carbs: 20g
- Fiber: 10g
- Protein: 5g

Beef and Veggie Hash

PREP TIME:
15 mins

COOKING TIME:
30 mins

SERVINGS:
2

INGREDIENTS:

- 1 lb ground beef
- 1 sweet potato, diced
- 1 bell pepper, diced
- 1/2 onion, diced
- 2 cloves garlic, minced
- 1 tbsp coconut oil
- 1/4 cup beef broth
- 1 tsp dried oregano

INSTRUCTIONS:

1. Preheat oven to 400°F.
2. In a skillet, brown beef over med-high heat. Transfer to plate.
3. In same pan, saute veggies in coconut oil until tender.
4. Return beef to pan. Add broth and oregano. Toss to combine.
5. Transfer to baking sheet. Roast 20-25 mins, stirring once until browned.

Nutritional Facts (per serving):

- Calories: 240
- Fat: 10g
- Carbs: 15g
- Fiber: 3g
- Protein: 25g

AIP Waffles

PREP TIME:
10 mins

COOKING TIME:
20 mins

SERVINGS:
4 waffles

INGREDIENTS:

- 2 bananas, mashed
- 1 cup arrowroot flour
- 1/4 cup coconut flour
- 1/2 tsp baking soda
- Pinch of unrefined salt (such as Himalayan Pink or Celtic Grey Salt)
- 1 tbsp coconut butter
- 1 cup coconut milk

INSTRUCTIONS:

1. In a bowl, mix the mashed banana with nut butter until combined.
2. In a separate bowl, whisk together the dry ingredients.
3. Add the dry ingredients to the wet and stir just to combine.
4. Fold in the coconut milk until a smooth batter forms.
5. Cook batter in a preheated waffle iron according to manufacturer's instructions.
6. Top waffles with extra nut butter. Enjoy!

Nutritional Facts (per waffle):

- Calories: 200
- Fat: 8g
- Carbs: 30g
- Fiber: 6g
- Protein: 4g

Turkey Sausage and Squash Bake

PREP TIME:	COOKING TIME:	SERVINGS:
15 mins	45 mins	2

INGREDIENTS:

- 1/3 lb turkey sausage links
- 1/3 butternut squash, peeled and cubed
- 1/3 onion, diced
- 1 clove garlic, minced
- 1 tbsp olive oil
- 1/3 tsp dried thyme
- 1 tbsp + 1 tsp chicken broth

INSTRUCTIONS:

1. Preheat oven to 375°F.
2. In a skillet over medium heat, brown sausage links. Slice each link into 3 pieces.
3. Transfer sausage to a baking dish. Toss with squash, onion, garlic and olive oil.
4. Pour chicken broth over ingredients and sprinkle with thyme.
5. Cover with foil and bake 30 mins. Uncover and bake 15 mins more until squash is tender.

Nutritional Facts (per serving):

- Calories: 110
- Fat: 4.5g
- Carbs: 9g
- Fiber: 2g
- Protein: 7g

Tropical Smoothie

PREP TIME:	COOKING TIME:	SERVINGS:
5 mins	None	2 smoothies

INGREDIENTS:

- 1 cup frozen banana slices
- 1 cup frozen mango chunks
- 1 cup fresh pineapple chunks
- 1 cup coconut milk

INSTRUCTIONS:

1. Add all ingredients to a high-powered blender.
2. Blend on high speed until smooth and creamy, about 2 minutes.
3. Pour into glasses filled with ice if desired.
4. Serve and enjoy!

Nutritional Facts (per smoothie):

- Calories: 300
- Fat: 15g
- Carbs: 45g
- Fiber: 7g
- Protein: 3g

Leftover Meat and Veggie Fritters

PREP TIME:	**COOKING TIME:**	**SERVINGS:**
15 mins	15 mins	6 fritters

INGREDIENTS:

- 1 cup leftover roasted veggies, chopped
- 1/2 cup leftover cooked meat, chopped
- 3 tbsp gelatin mixed with 9 tbsp water
- 1/4 cup coconut flakes
- 1 tbsp coconut oil

INSTRUCTIONS:

1. In a bowl, mix veggies and meat with gelatin mixture until combined.
2. Form into 6 patties and dust lightly with coconut flakes.
3. In a skillet over medium heat, heat coconut oil.
4. Cook fritters until golden brown, 3-4 minutes per side.
5. Drain on paper towel. Enjoy!

Nutritional Facts (per fritter):

- Calories: 70
- Fat: 4g
- Carbs: 2g
- Fiber: 1g
- Protein: 5g

Veggie Muffins

PREP TIME:
15 mins

COOKING TIME:
15 mins

SERVINGS:
6 muffins

INGREDIENTS:

- 3 tbsp gelatin mixed with 9 tbsp water
- 1/4 cup coconut milk
- 1/4 cup shredded vegetable cheese
- 2 tbsp ghee, divided
- Toppings of choice (spinach, tomato, onion, etc)

INSTRUCTIONS:

1. Preheat oven to 325°F. Line a muffin tin with paper liners.
2. In a bowl, mix gelatin mixture and milk until blended. Stir in vegetable cheese.
3. Melt 1 tbsp ghee in each liner. Pour in gelatin mixture until 2/3 full.
4. Bake for 15 mins until fully set. Add toppings before serving.

Nutritional Facts (per muffin):

- Calories: 80
- Fat: 6g
- Carbs: 0g
- Fiber: 0g
- Protein: 6g

Lox and Greens Salad

PREP TIME:	COOKING TIME:	SERVINGS:
15 mins	None	2

INGREDIENTS:

- 3 oz lox (smoked salmon)
- 2 cups mixed greens
- 1 avocado, diced
- 1 cucumber, diced
- 1/4 red onion, thinly sliced
- 2 tbsp olive oil
- 2 tbsp apple cider vinegar

INSTRUCTIONS:

1. In a large bowl, combine greens, avocado, cucumber and onion.
2. In a small jar, shake olive oil and vinegar to emulsify dressing.
3. Top salad with lox. Drizzle with dressing. Toss gently to combine.
4. Serve immediately. Enjoy!

Nutritional Facts (per serving):

- Calories: 170
- Fat: 13g
- Carbs: 6g
- Fiber: 4g
- Protein: 8g

Chicken Salad Lettuce Wraps

PREP TIME:	**COOKING TIME:**	**SERVINGS:**
15 mins	None	2

INGREDIENTS:

- 1 cup shredded cooked chicken
- 1/4 cup mayonnaise
- 1 tbsp diced celery
- 1 tbsp diced red onion
- 1/2 tsp lemon juice
- 4 lettuce leaves

INSTRUCTIONS:

1. In a bowl, mix chicken, mayonnaise, celery, onion and lemon juice until well combined.
2. Place about 1/4 cup chicken salad in the centre of each lettuce leaf.
3. Fold in sides and roll up tightly to encase filling.
4. Serve wraps and enjoy!

Nutritional Facts (per 2 wraps):

- Calories: 150
- Fat: 8g
- Carbs: 3g
- Fiber: 1g
- Protein: 16g

Ham and Pear Bowl

PREP TIME:	COOKING TIME:	SERVINGS:
15 mins	None .	2

INGREDIENTS:

- 2 cups mixed greens
- 1 pear, sliced
- 4 oz thinly sliced ham
- 1/4 cup shredded vegetable cheese
- 2 tbsp chopped coconut flakes in granola or trail mix
- 2 tbsp apple cider vinaigrette

INSTRUCTIONS:

1. Divide mixed greens between two bowls.
2. Top with pear slices, ham slices and shredded vegetable cheese.
3. Sprinkle coconut flakes (granola or trail mix) over top.
4. Drizzle vinaigrette over salads.
5. Toss lightly to coat. Enjoy!

Nutritional Fcts (per serving):

- Calories: 250
- Fat: 14g
- Carbs: 17g
- Fiber: 5g
- Protein: 18g

Breakfast Casserole

PREP TIME:	COOKING TIME:	SERVINGS:
15 mins	45 mins	2

INGREDIENTS:

- 1 small spaghetti squash
- 1 tablespoon coconut oil, divided
- 1/3 of 10-oz pack of frozen spinach
- 1/3 large onion, chopped
- 1 carrot, diced
- 1 celery stalk, diced
- 1/3 lb ground pork
- ½ of an 8-oz packs mushrooms, sliced
- 1 large zucchini, chopped
- 2 tablespoons chopped fresh sage
- 2 tablespoons chopped fresh rosemary
- ½ teaspoon dried thyme
- ½ teaspoon cinnamon
- ½ teaspoon onion powder
- ½ teaspoons sea salt
- ½ cup bone broth and/or coconut milk

INSTRUCTIONS:

1. Preheat the oven to 400°F (200°C). Cut the spaghetti squash in half lengthwise, scoop out the seeds, and place cut side down on a lined baking sheet. Roast for 45-50 minutes until tender. Use a fork to shred the squash into strands. Set aside.

2. Microwave the frozen spinach, drain excess liquid, and set aside.

3. In a large skillet, heat 1 tablespoon of coconut oil over medium heat. Sauté onion, carrots, and celery for 4-5 minutes until softened. Add ground pork and cook until browned. Stir in fresh herbs, spices, and salt.

4. In another skillet, heat the remaining coconut oil and sauté mushrooms and zucchini until softened, about 8 minutes. Stir in the cooked spinach.

5. Combine the contents of both skillets. Adjust seasoning with salt or herbs as needed.

6. Preheat the oven to 375°F (190°C). Grease a 9x13" baking dish. Stir the spaghetti squash into the skillet mixture and transfer everything to the baking dish. Pour bone broth and/or coconut milk evenly over the top.

7. Bake for 40-45 minutes until bubbly and the top is golden brown. Allow to cool slightly before serving.

Nutritional Facts (per serving):

- Calories: 250
- Fat: 15g
- Carbs: 5g
- Fiber: 1g
- Protein: 22g

Chapter 6

VEGETARIAN AND VEGAN AIP RECIPES

While meat and seafood provide valuable protein and nutrients for healing, going vegetarian or vegan can still be healthy and balanced on the Autoimmune Protocol if done correctly. This chapter showcases recipes for those seeking to limit or omit animal products while following AIP guidelines. You'll be pleasantly surprised at the variety of satisfying meals that can be created, from grain-free dips and snacks to hearty stew and chili recipes. Whether meat-free part or full-time, this selection of vegetarian and vegan options proves the AIP diet can easily accommodate different lifestyles and food preferences.

Rainbow Salad with Apple Cider Vinaigrette

PREP TIME:	COOKING TIME:	SERVINGS:
15 minutes	None	2

INGREDIENTS:

- 3 cups mixed greens
- 1 carrot, julienned
- 1/2 cucumber, diced
- 1 avocado, diced
- 1 apple, julienned
- Apple Cider Vinaigrette (recipe below)

Apple Cider Vinaigrette:

- 1/4 cup apple cider vinegar
- 1/2 shallot, minced
- 1 clove garlic, minced
- 1/2 cup olive oil
- 2 tbsp apple cider
- 1 tsp Dijon mustard
- Pinch of unrefined salt (such as Himalayan Pink or Celtic Grey Salt)

INSTRUCTIONS:

1. Make the vinaigrette by whisking together the apple cider vinegar, shallot, garlic, olive oil, apple cider, Dijon mustard, salt. Set aside.
2. In a large bowl, gently toss together the mixed greens, carrot, cucumber, avocado and apple.
3. Drizzle the vinaigrette over the salad and toss to coat evenly.
4. Serve immediately.

Nutritional Facts (per serving):

- Calories: 200
- Fat: 15g
- Carbs: 13g
- Fiber: 5g
- Protein: 3g

Turmeric Soup

PREP TIME:	COOKING TIME:	SERVINGS:
15 minutes	1 hour	2

INGREDIENTS:

- 2 cups bone broth or water
- 2 carrots, diced
- 1 small head cauliflower, chopped
- 2 cloves garlic, minced
- 1 tbsp coconut oil
- 1/2 tsp ground turmeric
- Pinch of unrefined salt (such as Himalayan Pink or Celtic Grey Salt)

INSTRUCTIONS:

1. In a large pot, heat the coconut oil over medium. Add the garlic and cook for 1 minute.
2. Add the broth, carrots, cauliflower, turmeric, salt. Bring to a boil.
3. Once boiling, reduce heat and simmer for 45-60 minutes.
4. Use an immersion blender to puree the soup slightly until creamy but still chunky.
5. Taste and adjust seasoning as needed. Serve warm.

Nutritional Facts (per serving):

- Calories: 180
- Fat: 2g
- Carbs: 30g
- Fiber: 12g
- Protein: 12g

Mushroom and Kale Sauté

PREP TIME:	COOKING TIME:	SERVINGS:
10 minutes	15 minutes	2

INGREDIENTS:

- 1/2 tbsp coconut oil or ghee
- 8 oz cremini or button mushrooms, sliced
- 1 bunch kale, thick stems removed, chopped
- 2 cloves garlic, minced
- Pinch of unrefined salt (such as Himalayan Pink or Celtic Grey Salt)

INSTRUCTIONS:

1. In a large skillet, heat the coconut oil over medium-high.
2. Add the mushrooms and cook for 5-7 minutes until browned, stirring occasionally.
3. Add the kale and garlic. Cook for 2-3 minutes until kale begins to wilt, stirring frequently.
4. Reduce heat to low, cover and cook for 5 more minutes until kale is tender.
5. Season with salt.
6. Serve warm.

Nutritional Facts (per serving):

- Calories: 50
- Fat: 2.5g
- Carbs: 5g
- Fiber: 2g
- Protein: 3g

Beet Chips

PREP TIME:	COOKING TIME:	SERVINGS:
10 minutes	50 minutes	2

INGREDIENTS:

- 0.88 pound raw beet
- 1 tablespoon olive oil
- Pinch of unrefined salt (such as Himalayan Pink or Celtic Grey Salt)

INSTRUCTIONS:

1. Preheating the oven to 302°F (150°C).
2. Beet should be peeled. To ensure that all of the dirt is gone, give it a good rinse in cold water. Finely slice it to a thickness of about 1 mm using a mandolin slicer (you can, technically, use a knife, but it will be more difficult).
3. Spread some oil on a baking sheet and line it with beet slices. Add a dash of salt and a drizzle of olive oil.
4. Bake for 50 to 60 minutes, or until the beetroot slices are crispy, after placing the baking sheet in the oven.

Nutritional Facts (per serving):

- Calories: 151
- Fat: 8g
- Carbs: 19g
- Fiber: 6g
- Protein: 3g

Spicy Roasted Roots

PREP TIME:

15 minutes

COOKING TIME:

40 minutes

SERVINGS:

2

INGREDIENTS:

- 1 beet, peeled and cut into 1-inch wedges
- 1 large turnip, peeled and cut into 1-inch pieces
- 1 large sweet potato, peeled and cut into 1-inch pieces
- 2 parsnips, peeled and cut into 1-inch pieces
- 2 tbsp olive oil
- 1 tsp dried thyme
- 1/2 tsp dried sage
- Pinch of unrefined salt (such as Himalayan Pink or Celtic Grey Salt)

INSTRUCTIONS:

1. Preheat oven to 400°F.
2. On a large baking sheet, toss the beet wedges, turnips, sweet potato and parsnips with the olive oil, thyme, sage, and salt until evenly coated.
3. Roast for 35-40 minutes, flipping halfway, until tender and lightly browned.
4. Serve warm. Enjoy!

Nutritional Facts (per serving):

- Calories: 140
- Fat: 5g
- Carbs: 25g
- Fiber: 6g
- Protein: 2g

Carrot Ginger Bisque

PREP TIME:	COOKING TIME:	SERVINGS:
15 minutes	30 minutes	2

INGREDIENTS:

- 1 lb carrots, peeled and chopped
- 2 leeks, white and light green parts sliced
- 1 tbsp coconut oil
- 2 cloves garlic, minced
- 1 tbsp grated ginger
- 4 cups bone broth or water
- 1/4 cup full fat coconut milk
- Salt and pepper to taste

INSTRUCTIONS:

1. In a saucepan, heat the coconut oil over medium. Cook the leeks for 5 minutes until softened.
2. Add the carrots, garlic and ginger. Sauté for 2 more minutes.
3. Pour in the bone broth and bring to a boil. Cover and simmer for 20 minutes, until carrots are very soft.
4. Allow to cool slightly. Working in batches, transfer soup to a high-powered blender and puree until smooth and creamy.
5. Return soup to pot and stir in coconut milk. Season with salt and pepper.
6. Serve warm, garnished with extra coconut milk if desired.

Nutritional Facts (per serving):

- Calories: 120
- Fat: 6g
- Carbs: 17g
- Fiber: 5g
- Protein: 3g

Lemon-Cilantro Roasted Brussels Sprouts

PREP TIME:	COOKING TIME:	SERVINGS:
5 minutes	30 mintues	2

INGREDIENTS:

- 1 pound Brussels sprouts, ends removed and quartered
- ⅓ cup avocado oil
- ½ bunch cilantro, chopped
- Zest and juice of ½ lemon
- Pinch of unrefined salt (such as Himalayan Pink or Celtic Grey Salt)

INSTRUCTIONS:

1. Preheat the oven to 425 degrees F (220°C).
2. Place the Brussels sprouts in a heavy-bottomed roasting pan, add avocado oil, and stir to combine. Bake for 10 minutes, then stir well. Continue baking for an additional 20 minutes without stirring, until sprouts are tender and browned.
3. Add chopped cilantro, lemon zest, lemon juice, and sea salt. Stir to combine thoroughly. Serve warm.

Nutritional Facts (per serving):

- Calories: 290
- Fat: 11g
- Carbs: 42g
- Fiber: 11g
- Protein: 11g

Sizzling Garlic Scapes

PREP TIME:	**COOK TIME:**	**SERVINGS:**
2 minutes	5 minutes	**2**

INGREDIENTS:

- ¼ - 1/2 lb green garlic scapes, cut into 3-inch pieces
- 2 tablespoons avocado, coconut, or olive oil
- Pinch of unrefined salt (such as Himalayan Pink or Celtic Grey Salt)
- Coconut aminos or lemon wedges, to garnish (optional)

INSTRUCTIONS:

1. Heat a medium cast iron or stainless steel skillet over medium-high heat with the oil until melted and shimmering.
2. Add the garlic scapes to the hot pan, season with salt, and toss to coat evenly with oil and salt.
3. Let the scapes cook undisturbed for 3-4 minutes until they develop deep colored blisters in spots. Adjust heat if needed to keep just below smoking.
4. Once the scapes are blistered, turn off the heat and toss them once more. The residual heat in the pan will finish cooking them to a crisp texture.
5. Garnish with a splash of coconut aminos or a squeeze of lemon juice before serving.

Nutritional Facts (per serving):

- Calories: 110
- Fat: 4g
- Carbs: 15g
- Fiber: 2g
- Protein: 4g

Vegetable Bibimbap

PREP TIME:	COOK TIME:	SERVINGS:
20 minutes	20 minutes	2

INGREDIENTS:

- 1 head cauliflower
- 1 zucchini, diced
- 8 shiitake mushrooms, stems removed and sliced
- 1 carrot, julienned
- 2 scallions, sliced
- 2 cloves garlic, minced
- 1 inch ginger, grated
- 3 tbsp coconut aminos or tamari

INSTRUCTIONS:

1. Grate cauliflower to make "rice" and place in a food processor. Pulse until rice-like consistency.
2. In a skillet over medium-high heat, sauté zucchini, mushrooms, carrot and scallions with garlic and ginger until tender. Remove from skillet.
3. To serve, portion cauliflower rice into bowls and top with vegetable mixture. Enjoy!

Nutrition Facts (per serving):

- Calories: 110
- Fat: 6g
- Carbs: 9g
- Fiber: 3g
- Protein: 8g

Butternut Squash Tacos

PREP TIME:	**COOK TIME:**	**SERVINGS:**
30 minutes	30 minutes	6

INGREDIENTS:

- 1/2 medium butternut squash, peeled and cubed
- 2 tbsp coconut oil
- 1 head green cabbage, shredded
- 1 carrot, grated
- 1 avocado, diced
- 4 collard green or cabbage leaves
- Lime wedges

INSTRUCTIONS:

1. Preheat oven to 400°F. Toss butternut squash with 1 tbsp coconut oil on a baking sheet. Roast for 30 minutes.
2. In a bowl, toss shredded cabbage and carrot with remaining 1 tbsp coconut oil.
3. To assemble, place roasted squash in center of collard green leaf. Top with cabbage slaw and avocado.
4. Serve with lime wedges to squeeze over tacos. Enjoy!

Nutritional Facts (per taco):

- Calories: 80
- Fat: 4g
- Carbs: 11g
- Fiber: 3g
- Protein: 2g

Cauliflower Steaks

PREP TIME:
10 minutes

COOK TIME:
25 minutes

SERVINGS:
2

INGREDIENTS:

- 1 small head cauliflower
- 2 tbsp ghee or coconut oil, melted
- 2 cloves garlic, minced
- 1 tsp dried thyme
- Pinch of unrefined salt (such as Himalayan Pink or Celtic Grey Salt)

INSTRUCTIONS:

1. Preheat oven to 400°F.
2. Cut cauliflower head into 1-inch thick slices through the core. You should get 4 large "steaks".
3. In a small bowl, mix melted ghee/oil with garlic, thyme and salt.
4. Place cauliflower steaks on a baking sheet. Brush tops generously with ghee mixture.
5. Roast for 20-25 minutes, brushing steaks with more ghee halfway, until tender and browned.
6. Serve warm. Enjoy!

Nutritional Facts (per serving):

- Calories: 70
- Fat: 5g
- Carbs: 6g
- Fiber: 3g
- Protein: 3g

Kohlrabi with Shiitake

PREP TIME:
15 minutes

COOK TIME:
15 minutes

SERVINGS:
2

INGREDIENTS:

- 1 kohlrabi, peeled and julienned
- 4 shiitake mushrooms, stems removed and sliced
- 1 scallion, sliced
- 1 clove garlic, minced
- 1 tablespoon ghee or coconut oil
- 1 tablespoon tamari or coconut aminos

INSTRUCTIONS:

1. In a large skillet, heat the ghee over medium-high. Add the kohlrabi and mushrooms and stir-fry for 5 minutes.
2. Push veggies to the sides.
3. Add the scallions, garlic and tamari. Stir-fry for 2 more minutes.
4. Enjoy!

Nutritional Facts (per serving):

- Calories: 80
- Fat: 4g
- Carbs: 7g
- Fiber: 3g
- Protein: 4g

Purple Potato Salad

PREP TIME:
15 minutes

COOK TIME:
15 minutes

SERVINGS:
2

INGREDIENTS:

- 1/2 lb small purple sweet potatoes
- 2 tbsp olive oil
- 2 tbsp fresh dill, chopped
- 2 tbsp capers, rinsed and chopped
- 1 tbsp apple cider vinegar
- Pinch of unrefined salt (such as Himalayan Pink or Celtic Grey Salt)

INSTRUCTIONS:

1. Place potatoes in a saucepan and cover with water. Bring to a boil and cook for 15 minutes, until tender when pierced with a fork.
2. Drain potatoes and allow to cool slightly. Cut into quarters if large.
3. In a large bowl, whisk together olive oil, dill, capers, vinegar and salt.
4. Add warm potatoes and toss gently to coat. Allow to marinate for 30 minutes before serving to absorb flavors.
5. Serve chilled or at room temperature. Enjoy!

Nutritional Facts (per serving):

- Calories: 90
- Fat: 4g
- Carbs: 13g
- Fiber: 2g
- Protein: 2g

Creamy Coconut Greens

PREP TIME:	COOK TIME:	SERVINGS:
15 minutes	20 minutes	4

INGREDIENTS:

- 2 tablespoons unsweetened coconut flakes
- 1 pound mixed hardy greens (such as Tuscan kale, curly kale, Swiss chard, and/or mustard greens; about 4 bunches); remove ribs and stems and discard; cut leaves into 1-inch strips
- 2 tablespoons coconut oil
- 3 garlic cloves, finely chopped
- 1/2 large onion, finely chopped
- 2-inch piece ginger, peeled and grated
- Pinch of unrefined salt (such as Himalayan Pink or Celtic Grey Salt)
- 1 teaspoon ganthoda powder
- 1/2 teaspoon ground turmeric
- 1 cup coconut milk

INSTRUCTIONS:

1. In a dry pan over high heat, toast coconut flakes for a few minutes until slightly browned. Remove from the pan and set aside.

2. Heat coconut oil in a large skillet over medium heat. Add garlic, onions, and ginger. Cook, stirring often, until onions are softened, about 5 minutes. Season with salt, then add ganthoda powder and turmeric. Stir to combine and cook for 1 more minute.

3. Pour coconut milk into the skillet and bring to a simmer. Add greens a handful at a time, allowing each handful to wilt slightly before adding more. Cook, tossing occasionally, until greens are tender and the mixture appears creamy, about 10 minutes.

4. Taste and adjust seasoning with more salt if necessary.

5. Transfer the creamy greens to a platter or large shallow bowl. Top with toasted coconut flakes and chopped cilantro before serving.

Nutrition Facts (per serving):

- Calories: 200
- Fat: 7g
- Carbs: 35g
- Fiber: 5g
- Protein: 3g

Tropical Green Blast

PREP TIME:
5 minutes

COOKING TIME:
None

SERVINGS:
2

INGREDIENTS:

- 1 cup coconut water
- 1 banana, frozen
- 1 cup baby spinach
- 1/2 avocado
- 1/2 cup mango, frozen
- 1/4 cup pineapple, frozen

INSTRUCTIONS:

1. Add all ingredients to a high-powered blender.
2. Blend on high speed until smooth and creamy, 1-2 minutes.
3. Pour into glasses and serve chilled.

Nutritional Facts (per serving):

- Calories: 180
- Fat: 8g
- Carbs: 30g
- Fiber: 7g
- Protein: 3g

Chapter 7

POULTRY, MEAT AND ORGAN MEAT AIP RECIPES

Protein plays an important role in the Autoimmune Protocol (AIP) diet as it provides essential amino acids and nutrients to support healing and immune function. This chapter focuses on recipes centered around high-quality, nutritious animal proteins like poultry, red meat and organ meats permitted on the AIP diet. Chicken, turkey, beef, lamb and organ meats such as liver are fully compliant protein options packed with vitamins, minerals and antioxidants to nourish the body during the elimination phase. The following recipes showcase creative ways to prepare and enjoy these proteins while avoiding common allergens and focusing on anti-inflammatory preparation methods like slow cooking. Whether as a main dish or addition to meals, these recipes will help ensure adequate protein intake on the AIP diet.

Slow Cooker Beef Stew

PREP TIME:
30 minutes

COOKING TIME:
8 hours

SERVINGS:
6

INGREDIENTS:

- 2/3 lb beef chuck, cubed
- 2 carrots, chopped
- 1 stalk celery, chopped
- 1/2 onion, chopped
- 1-2 cloves garlic, minced
- 1/3 cup red wine
- 1 1/3 cups beef bone broth
- 2 bay leaves
- 1 tsp thyme

INSTRUCTIONS:

1. Place beef in slow cooker. Top with carrots, celery, onion and garlic.
2. Pour in wine and bone broth. Add bay leaves and thyme.
3. Cover and cook on low heat for 8 hours, until meat is tender.
4. Discard bay leaves before serving. Season with your desired dressing.

Nutritional Facts (per serving):

- Calories: 230
- Fat: 8g
- Carbs: 8g
- Fiber: 2g
- Protein: 26g

Liver & Onions

PREP TIME:
15 minutes

COOKING TIME:
30 minutes

SERVINGS:
2

INGREDIENTS:

- 1/2 lb calf's liver, sliced
- 1 onion, sliced
- 2 cloves garlic, minced
- 1 tbsp ghee or avocado oil
- vegetables for serving

INSTRUCTIONS:

1. Slice onions and heat ghee in a skillet over medium. Cook onions until softened and browned, about 15 minutes.
2. Season liver slices with salt. Add to skillet and cook 3-5 minutes per side, until crispy around edges but still pink inside.
3. Serve liver and onions with veggies.

Nutritional Facts (per serving):

- Calories: 150
- Fat: 7g
- Carbs: 8g
- Fiber: 1g
- Protein: 16g

Herbed Lamb Chops

PREP TIME:	**COOKING TIME:**	**SERVINGS:**
5 minutes	15 minutes	2

INGREDIENTS:

- 4 lamb loin chops
- 1 clove garlic, minced
- 1 tbsp fresh rosemary, chopped
- 1 tbsp fresh thyme, chopped
- Salt to taste
- Olive oil

INSTRUCTIONS:

1. Season lamb chops liberally with salt, garlic, rosemary and thyme.
2. Heat olive oil in skillet over medium-high. Working in batches, cook chops 5-7 minutes per side for medium-rare doneness.
3. Allow to rest 5 minutes before serving.

Nutritional Facts (per serving):

- Calories: 300
- Fat: 18g
- Carbs: 1g
- Fiber: 0g
- Protein: 34g

Bacon Wrapped Pork Tenderloin

PREP TIME:	**COOKING TIME:**	**SERVINGS:**
10 minutes	30 minutes	2

INGREDIENTS:

- 0.5-0.75 lbs pork tenderloin
- 4 slices uncooked bacon
- Salt to taste

INSTRUCTIONS:

1. Season pork all over with salt. Wrap each slice of bacon around tenderloin, securing with toothpicks.
2. Roast on baking sheet at 400°F for 30 minutes, until internal temp reaches 160°F.
3. Remove toothpicks and slice pork. Discard rendered bacon fat if desired.

Nutritional Facts (per serving):

- Calories: 250
- Fat: 15g
- Carbs: 1g
- Fiber: 0g
- Protein: 26g

Grilled Chicken Wings with Homemade BBQ Sauce

PREP TIME:	COOKING TIME:	SERVINGS:
15 minutes	30 minutes	2

INGREDIENTS:

For the chicken wings marinade:

- About 1 lb chicken wings
- 1 tablespoon lemon juice
- 1/2 tablespoon garlic powder
- Pinch of unrefined salt (such as Himalayan Pink or Celtic Grey Salt)
- 1 tablespoon avocado oil

For the BBQ sauce:

- ¼ cup coconut aminos
- 2 tablespoons apple cider vinegar
- 1 tablespoon balsamic vinegar
- 1 teaspoon fresh grated ginger
- 1 tablespoon ground ginger
- 1 tablespoon honey
- 2 tablespoons unsulfured blackstrap molasses
- ½ teaspoon arrowroot starch mixed with 2 tablespoons water

INSTRUCTIONS:

Baking the chicken wings:

1. Preheat the oven to 425°F (220°C).
2. In a mixing bowl, combine all the marinade ingredients. Toss the chicken wings in the marinade until well coated.
3. Lightly brush a baking tray with avocado oil and arrange the wings on it.
4. Bake in the preheated oven for 20-22 minutes until the bottoms become crisp. Flip the wings and bake for an additional 5-7 minutes until fully cooked. Remove from the oven and keep covered until ready to serve.

Making the BBQ sauce:

5. While the wings are baking, prepare the sauce. In a saucepan over low heat,

combine all sauce ingredients except the arrowroot slurry. Stir with a whisk and allow the mixture to simmer for a couple of minutes.

6. Add the arrowroot starch mixed with water to the saucepan, whisking continuously until the sauce thickens, about 2 minutes. Remove from heat and let cool for 5 minutes.

Serving the wings:

7. Arrange the baked wings on a serving tray and pour the BBQ sauce over them. Use tongs to coat each wing evenly with sauce.

8. Serve immediately and enjoy your grilled chicken wings with homemade BBQ sauce!

Nutritional Facts:

- Calories: 60
- Fat: 3g
- Carbs: 2g
- Fiber: 0g
- Protein: 6g

Baked Meatballs

PREP TIME:	**COOKING TIME:**	**SERVINGS:**
15 minutes	30 minutes	2

INGREDIENTS:

- 1/3 lb ground beef
- 1/3 lb ground turkey
- Pinch of unrefined salt (such as Himalayan Pink or Celtic Grey Salt)
- 1/2 teaspoon AIP-friendly seasoning blend
- ½ cup portobello mushrooms, finely chopped and sautéed
- 1 tablespoon+1 teaspoon onion, finely chopped

INSTRUCTIONS:

1. Preheat the oven to 400°F (200°C).
2. In a large bowl, combine the ground beef, ground turkey, sea salt, AIP-friendly seasoning blend, sautéed portobello mushrooms, and chopped onion. Mix until well combined.
3. Using a scoop or your hands, form 1- to 2-inch sized meatballs and place them on a baking sheet.
4. Bake in the preheated oven for 15 to 20 minutes, or until the center of the meatballs reaches 160°F (71°C).
5. Remove from the oven and let them cool slightly before serving.
6. Enjoy your oven-baked meatballs!

Nutritional Facts:

- Calories: 150
- Fat: 6g
- Carbs: 10g
- Fiber: 3g
- Protein: 15g

Italian Sausage Soup

PREP TIME:
15 minutes

COOKING TIME:
30 minutes

SERVINGS:
2

INGREDIENTS:

- 1/3 lb Italian sausage links
- 1/2 onion, diced
- 1-2 cloves garlic, minced
- 2 cups chicken or bone broth
- 2 cups chopped kale

INSTRUCTIONS:

1. In soup pot over medium, brown sausage links. Remove from pot and slice into rounds.
2. Sauté onion and garlic in pot until softened.
3. Return sausage to pot. Add broth and kale. Simmer 20 minutes.

Nutritional Facts (per serving):

- Calories: 200
- Fat: 8g
- Carbs: 16g
- Fiber: 4g
- Protein: 15g

Chili Lime Flank Steak

PREP TIME:	COOKING TIME:	SERVINGS:
5 minutes	10 minutes	2

INGREDIENTS:

- 0.75 lbs flank steak
- 1 tbsp chili powder
- Zest of 1 lime
- Salt to taste
- Lime wedges

INSTRUCTIONS:

1. Rub steak all over with salt, chili powder and lime zest.
2. Heat skillet over high with 1 tbsp ghee or oil. Sear steak 3-4 minutes per side for medium-rare doneness.
3. Remove from heat and let stand 5 minutes.

Nutritional Facts (per serving):

- Calories: 230
- Fat: 11g
- Carbs: 1g
- Fiber: 0g
- Protein: 33g

Garlic Rosemary Rack of Lamb

PREP TIME:	COOKING TIME:	SERVINGS:
5 minutes	15 minutes	2

INGREDIENTS:

- 1/2 rack of lamb (4 chops)
- 1 clove garlic, minced
- 1 tbsp fresh rosemary, chopped
- Olive oil, salt

INSTRUCTIONS:

1. Season lamb all over with salt, rosemary and garlic.
2. Heat olive oil in oven-safe skillet over medium-high. Sear lamb 3-4 minutes per side.
3. Transfer skillet to oven and roast 10-12 minutes for medium-rare doneness.
4. Let rest 5 minutes before slicing between chops.

Nutritional Facts (per serving):

- Calories: 290
- Fat: 16g
- Carbs: 1g
- Fiber: 0g
- Protein: 36g

Protein Power Bowl

PREP TIME:	COOKING TIME:	SERVINGS:
5 minutes	20 minutes	2

INGREDIENTS:

For the lamb:

- 1/2 cup Dijon mustard (omit for AIP)
- Juice of 1 whole lemon, plus lemon rinds saved
- 1 pound boneless lamb leg
- 1 cup bone broth

Salad add-ins (OPTIONAL):

- Pickled onions (store-bought or homemade)
- 1 small cucumber, sliced
- 1 bag cauliflower rice, cooked
- 4 cups mixed greens
- Olive oil and lemon (for dressing)

INSTRUCTIONS:

1. Preheat the oven to 325°F (160°C).
2. Place the lamb on a roasting rack or a baking sheet if you don't have a rack. Pour bone broth over the lamb. Rub Dijon mustard all over the lamb, then squeeze the lemon juice over it. Place the lemon rinds on top. Cover the pan with foil.
3. Bake the lamb for 2 hours, then flip it and cook for an additional 2 hours, covered, until the lamb is tender and easily shreds with two forks. Remove from the oven and shred the lamb. Set aside.
4. While the lamb is cooking, prepare optional cauliflower rice and any additional salad ingredients you prefer.
5. To assemble the power bowl, divide mixed greens among serving bowls. Top with shredded lamb, optional cauliflower rice, sliced cucumber, and pickled onions.
6. Drizzle with olive oil and lemon juice, or your preferred dressing.
7. Enjoy your Shredded Lamb Power Bowl!

Nutritional Facts (per serving):

- Calories: 400
- Fat: 15g
- Carbs: 32g
- Fiber: 8g
- Protein: 35g

Ginger Chicken Meatballs

PREP TIME:
15 minutes

COOKING TIME:
20 minutes

SERVINGS:
2

INGREDIENTS:

- 1/3 lb ground chicken
- 1 scallion, minced
- 1/2 clove garlic, minced
- 1 teaspoon grated ginger
- 2 tablespoons + 2 teaspoons coconut flakes
- Soy sauce or coconut aminos to taste

INSTRUCTIONS:

1. Preheat oven to 400°F. Line baking sheet with parchment paper.
2. In a bowl, mix chicken, scallions, garlic, ginger, coconut flakes, and soy sauce until well combined.
3. Roll mixture into 1-inch balls and place on prepared baking sheet.
4. Bake for 20 minutes, flipping once, until cooked through and lightly browned.

Nutritional Facts (per serving):

- Calories: 50
- Fat: 2g
- Carbs: 1g
- Fiber: 0g
- Protein: 7g

Citrus Chicken Kebabs

PREP TIME:	COOKING TIME:	SERVINGS:
15 minutes	12 minutes	2

INGREDIENTS:

- 1/2 lb chicken breast, cut into cubes
- 1/2 orange, zested and juiced
- 1 sprig fresh thyme, chopped
- 1 teaspoon ghee or olive oil
- Vegetable skewers

INSTRUCTIONS:

1. Toss chicken cubs with orange zest, juice and thyme. Thread onto skewers.
2. Heat grill or broiler. Brush kebabs with ghee.
3. Grill or broil 5-6 minutes per side until chicken is fully cooked.

Nutritional Facts (per serving):

- Calories: 110
- Fat: 2g
- Carbs: 2g
- Fiber: 0g
- Protein: 21g

Turkey Cranberry Wrap

PREP TIME:
5 minutes

COOKING TIME:
15 minutes

SERVINGS:
4 wraps

INGREDIENTS:

- 4 collard green leaves
- 2 cups cooked and shredded turkey or chicken
- 1 avocado, thinly sliced
- 2 cups roasted squash or sweet potato, cooked and sliced or mashed

CRANBERRY DATE SAUCE INGREDIENTS:

- 7.5 ounce container (2 cups) fresh cranberries
- 5 dates, finely chopped
- 5 basil leaves, thinly sliced
- ¼ teaspoon cinnamon
- ¼ cup water
- ¼ cup cold-pressed apple juice

INSTRUCTIONS:

1. In a saucepan over medium heat, combine cranberries, dates, basil, cinnamon, water, and apple juice.
2. Simmer, stirring occasionally, until cranberries burst and the mixture thickens. Set aside to cool.
3. Bring a large pan of water to a boil, then reduce heat to low.
4. Dip each collard green leaf into the hot water for about 5 seconds on each side to soften. Remove and drain.
5. Trim the tough stems and shave down the midrib of each leaf to ease folding.
6. Lay a collard green leaf flat. Along the midrib, spread cranberry date sauce, roasted squash or sweet potato, avocado slices, and shredded turkey or chicken.
7. Fold the sides of the leaf towards the center, then roll tightly from one end to create a wrap.
8. Optionally, slice the wraps before serving. Enjoy your Harvest Wrap with Cranberry Date Sauce, a delicious way to enjoy post-Thanksgiving flavors!

Nutritional Facts (per serving):

- Calories: 110
- Fat: 3g
- Carbs: 5g
- Fiber: 2g
- Protein: 15g

Beef & Broccoli Stir Fry

PREP TIME:

15 minutes

COOKING TIME:

10 minutes

SERVINGS:

2

INGREDIENTS:

- 6 oz beef flank steak
- 1/2 head broccoli, florets
- 2 cloves garlic, minced
- 1 tablespoon coconut aminos or tamari

INSTRUCTIONS:

1. Slice steak against grain into strips.
2. Stir fry steak and broccoli with garlic in coconut aminos 2-3 minutes.
3. Serve over cauli rice or alone.

Nutritional Facts (per serving):

- Calories: 160
- Fat: 5g
- Carbs: 5g
- Fiber: 2g
- Protein: 23g

Grilled Chicken Thighs

PREP TIME:	COOKING TIME:	SERVINGS:
15 minutes	30 minutes	2

INGREDIENTS:

For the chicken:

- Pinch of unrefined salt (such as Himalayan Pink or Celtic Grey Salt)
- ½ teaspoon ginger powder
- ½ teaspoon garlic powder
- 1.5 pounds bone-in, skin-on chicken thighs

For the salsa:

- ½ large pineapple, cut into ½-inch chunks
- 1 bunch radishes, tops removed and cut into ½-inch chunks
- 1 medium cucumber, cut into ½-inch chunks
- 1 avocado, cut into ½-inch chunks
- 1 bunch green onions, roots and top ends removed, finely chopped
- 1 ounce fresh mint leaves, finely chopped
- 1 clove garlic, minced
- ½ teaspoon sea salt
- ½ teaspoon ginger powder
- Juice of ½ lemon

INSTRUCTIONS:

1. In a small bowl, combine sea salt, ginger powder, and garlic powder.
2. Pat dry the chicken thighs with paper towels and set aside.
3. Just before grilling, rub the spice mixture evenly over the chicken thighs.
4. Place the chicken thighs skin-side down on the hot grill.
5. Grill for 5-7 minutes until the skin starts to crisp. Flip and grill for another 5-7 minutes, or until the internal temperature reaches 165°F (75°C).
6. In a mixing bowl, combine pineapple, radishes, cucumber, avocado, green onions, mint leaves, garlic, sea salt, ginger powder, and lemon juice. Gently stir to combine.

7. Serve each grilled chicken thigh topped with pineapple-mint salsa.

8. Enjoy your Grilled Chicken Thighs with Pineapple-Mint Salsa!

Nutritional Facts:

- Calories: 340
- Fat: 16g
- Carbs: 6g
- Fiber: 3g
- Protein: 39g

Chapter 8

FISH AND SHELLFISH AIP RECIPES

Seafood is an extremely nutritious protein for the AIP diet, providing an abundance of anti-inflammatory omega-3 fatty acids while being low in carbohydrates. Unlike red meat or poultry, many fish and shellfish varieties can be easily digested and are considered highly compliant on the elimination phase. From mild whitefish to robust salmon, this chapter features recipes that highlight the versatility and health benefits of a variety of compliant fish and shellfish. With preparation methods like baking, poaching and stir-frying, these dishes are simple to make yet richly flavored and satisfying. Including more fish and seafood meals is an excellent way to boost nutrient intake while supporting the healing goals of the AIP protocol. The following recipes will help you enjoy a variety of nutrient-dense seafood in tasty, compliant dishes.

Salmon Cakes with Remoulade Sauce

PREP TIME:
15 minutes

COOKING TIME:
10 minutes

SERVINGS:
2

INGREDIENTS:

- ½ lb salmon fillet, cooked and flaked
- 1/2 cup coconut flakes
- 2 Tbsp each fresh dill, minced onion
- 1/2 cup remoulade sauce

INSTRUCTIONS:

1. Mix salmon, coconut flakes, herbs and onion. Form 4 patties.
2. Pan fry patties until golden brown. Serve with remoulade sauce.

Nutritional Facts (per patty):

- Calories: 150
- Fat: 8g
- Carbs: 2g
- Fiber: 1g
- Protein: 16g

Shrimp and Grits

PREP TIME:
15 minutes

COOKING TIME:
20 minutes

SERVINGS:
2

INGREDIENTS:

- 1/2 lb shrimp, peeled
- 1/2 onion, diced
- 2 cloves garlic, minced
- 1 tbsp ghee
- 2 cups chicken broth
- 1/2 cup polenta or grits
- 1 green onion, sliced

INSTRUCTIONS:

1. Bring broth to boil, whisk in grits. Reduce heat and simmer 15 mins.
2. Sauté shrimp, onion and garlic until shrimp are pink.
3. Stir into cooked grits. Top with green onion.

Nutritional Facts (per serving):

- Calories: 250
- Fat: 5g
- Carbs: 30g
- Fiber: 2g
- Protein: 22g

Tuna Poke Bowls

PREP TIME:

15 minutes

SERVINGS:

2

INGREDIENTS:

- 1/2 lb ahi tuna, diced
- 1 avocado, diced
- 1/2 cup shredded cabbage
- 1 carrot, julienned
- 1 tsp toasted sesame oil
- 2 Tbsp ginger sauce
- Scallions

INSTRUCTIONS:

1. Divide ingredients among bowls: tuna, avocado, cabbage, carrot.
2. Drizzle with sesame oil and ginger sauce. Top with scallions.

Nutritional Facts (per serving):

- Calories: 200
- Fat: 9g
- Carbs: 7g
- Fiber: 4g
- Protein: 24g

Poached Whole Snapper

PREP TIME:	COOKING TIME:	SERVINGS:
10 minutes	15 minutes	2

INGREDIENTS:

- 1 (1lb) whole red snapper, gutted
- 1/2 onion, sliced
- 1 carrot, sliced
- 1 celery stalk, sliced
- 1/2 cup white wine
- Herb ramekins

INSTRUCTIONS:

1. Place fish and veggies in pot. Add wine and water to cover.
2. Poach gently until flesh flakes, about 15 min. Serve fillets with sauce.

Nutritional Facts (per serving):

- Calories: 150
- Fat: 3g
- Carbs: 3g
- Fiber: 1g
- Protein: 26g

Cod en Papillote

PREP TIME:
15 minutes

COOKING TIME:
15 minutes

SERVINGS:
2

INGREDIENTS:

- 1 tablespoon olive oil
- 2 small zucchini, sliced
- ½ cup chopped cilantro
- ½ cup chopped parsley
- 2 green onions, chopped
- 2 sprigs fresh thyme (or 2 teaspoons dried thyme)
- 1 lemon, thinly sliced
- 2 filets of haddock or other white fish
- Pinch of unrefined salt (such as Himalayan Pink or Celtic Grey Salt)

INSTRUCTIONS:

1. Preheat the oven to 400°F (200°C).
2. Cut two pieces of parchment paper into squares, each twice as big as the fish filets.
3. Fold each piece of parchment in half and cut out a half-heart shape (so when unfolded, it forms a heart shape).
4. Lay each parchment heart on a baking sheet.
5. Divide the sliced zucchini and lemon slices evenly onto each parchment heart, placing them in the center.
6. Place one filet of fish on top of the zucchini and lemon on each parchment.
7. Season each fish filet with sea salt.
8. Top each filet with additional lemon slices, cilantro, parsley, green onions, and thyme.
9. Fold over the edges of the parchment paper to cover the fish and herbs.
10. Starting from one end, tightly fold the open edge of the paper to seal the packets securely.
11. Place the packets on the baking sheet in the oven and bake for 10-12 minutes, until the fish is cooked through and flakes easily with a fork.
12. Carefully transfer each parchment packet to a plate.

13. Open the packets at the table to release the aromatic steam and serve immediately.

Nutritional Facts (per serving):

- Calories: 180
- Fat: 6g
- Carbs: 10g
- Fiber: 2g
- Protein: 21g

Scallop and Zucchini Skewers

PREP TIME:	**COOKING TIME:**	**SERVINGS:**
15 minutes	8 minutes	2

INGREDIENTS:

- 1/2 lb scallops
- 1 zucchini, quartered
- 4 basil leaves
- 1Tbsp ghee or coconut oil

INSTRUCTIONS:

1. Alternate scallops, zucchini and basil on skewers.
2. Brush with ghee and season. Grill or broil until scallops opaque.

Nutritional Facts (per skewer):

- Calories: 110
- Fat: 4.5g
- Carbs: 4g
- Fiber: 1g
- Protein: 14g

Honey-Citrus Glazed Arctic Char

PREPARATION TIME:	COOKING TIME:	SERVES:
35 minutes	18 minutes	2

INGREDIENTS:

For the Fish:

- 1 lb arctic char (approximately 2-3 fillets)
- Sea salt to taste

For the Glaze:

- 1/2 cup coconut-derived soy alternative
- 2-2 1/2 teaspoons fresh orange juice
- 1/4 - 1/3 cup pure maple syrup
- 1 tablespoon unfiltered apple vinegar
- 2 teaspoons minced fresh garlic
- 1 teaspoon grated fresh ginger
- Pinch of sea salt
- 1/2 teaspoon tapioca starch

Optional Garnish:

- Chopped scallions
- Fresh cilantro leaves

INSTRUCTIONS:

1. In a small saucepan, combine all glaze ingredients except the tapioca starch.
2. Gently heat the mixture, whisking to incorporate, until it reaches a gentle boil.
3. Reduce heat to low and simmer for about 5 minutes to concentrate flavors.
4. Gradually add tapioca starch, stirring constantly until the sauce thickens slightly.
5. Remove from heat and allow to cool to room temperature.
6. While cooling, prepare the arctic char by seasoning with sea salt.
7. Place fish in a sealed container with 1/3 of the cooled glaze. Refrigerate for 30 minutes (or overnight for deeper flavor).
8. Heat a large skillet over medium-high heat with a small amount of oil.

9. Cook marinated arctic char for 3-5 minutes per side, or until it reaches an internal temperature of 145°F.
10. Drizzle additional glaze over the cooked fish as desired.
11. Serve immediately with your choice of accompaniments.

Nutritional Values (per serving, approximate):

- Calories: 380
- Protein: 28g
- Fat: 22g
- Carbohydrates: 18g
- Fiber: 0g
- Sugar: 16g
- Sodium: 580mg

Shrimp and Mango Rice Bowl

PREP TIME:
30 minutes

SERVINGS:
2

INGREDIENTS:

- Cauliflower rice, prepared and seasoned to taste (or microwavable cauliflower rice for convenience)
- Sliced cucumbers
- Mango, sliced into small pieces
- Sliced or chopped avocado
- 1/2 lb shrimp, peeled, deveined, boiled, and sliced
- Roasted garlic granules or powder (plain garlic powder can be used)
- Sea salt

Garnishes:

- Sliced purple cabbage
- Sliced green onions
- AIP-friendly seaweed
- Lime wedges

Dipping Sauce:

- Coconut aminos
- A splash of lime juice
- Honey, to taste (or substitute with teriyaki sauce)

INSTRUCTIONS:

1. Prepare small to medium-sized bowls. Start with cauliflower rice as the base and season with roasted garlic seasoning and sea salt to your liking.
2. Arrange shrimp, cucumbers, mango, and avocado over the cauliflower rice.
3. Add garnishes such as sliced purple cabbage, green onions, and AIP-friendly seaweed.
4. Drizzle or dip with your preferred sauce and serve immediately.

Nutritional Facts (per serving):

- Calories: 150
- Fat: 7g
- Carbs: 5g
- Fiber: 3g
- Protein: 17g

Baked Halibut with Herb Vinaigrette

PREP TIME:	COOKING TIME:	SERVINGS:
10 minutes	15 minutes	2

INGREDIENTS:

- 2 (3 oz) halibut fillets
- 1/2 shallot, minced
- 1 tablespoon olive oil
- 1 Tbsp red wine vinegar
- 1/4 cup fresh herbs
- Salt

INSTRUCTIONS:

1. Season fish with salt. Place in baking dish.
2. Whisk shallot, oil, vinegar and herbs. Spread over fillets.
3. Bake 15 minutes until fish flakes. Serve drizzled with pan sauce.

Nutritional Facts (per fillet):

- Calories: 300
- Fat: 16g
- Carbs: 1g
- Fiber: 0g
- Protein: 39g

Caesar Salad with Roasted Salmon

PREP TIME:	COOKING TIME:	SERVINGS:
10 minutes	15 minutes	2

INGREDIENTS:

- 1/2 lb salmon fillet
- 1/2 head romaine lettuce
- 2 tablespoons Caesar dressing
- 2 tablespoons pine nuts
- Lemon wedges

INSTRUCTIONS:

1. Roast salmon at 400°F until flaky, about 15 minutes.
2. Chop romaine, top with salmon, dressing and pine nuts. Serve with lemon.

Nutritional Facts (per serving):

- Calories: 330
- Fat: 22g
- Carbs: 4g
- Fiber: 2g
- Protein: 27g

Seared Tuna Salad

PREP TIME:
10 minutes

COOKING TIME:
5 minutes

SERVINGS:
2

INGREDIENTS:

- 1/2 lb tuna steaks
- 2 cups mixed greens
- 1 avocado, diced
- 1 carrot, julienned
- Ginger vinaigrette

INSTRUCTIONS:

1. Season tuna with salt and pepper. Sear in hot skillet until outer edges are opaque, 1-2 minutes per side.
2. Chop seared tuna and toss with mixed greens, avocado and carrot. Drizzle with vinaigrette.

Nutritional Facts (per serving):

- Calories: 230
- Fat: 11g
- Carbs: 7g
- Fiber: 4g
- Protein: 28g

Shellfish Boil

PREP TIME:	**COOKING TIME:**	**SERVINGS:**
15 minutes	10 minutes	2

INGREDIENTS:

- 1/2 lb shrimp, peeled
- 6 mussels, debearded
- 6 red potatoes (sweet)
- 2 baby carrots
- 1/2 onion, quartered
- Fish broth

INSTRUCTIONS:

1. Add all ingredients to a pot and cover with broth.
2. Steam over medium until potatoes are tender and mussels open.

Nutritional Facts (per serving):

- Calories: 200
- Fat: 2g
- Carbs: 25g
- Fiber: 3g
- Protein: 20g

Mahi Mahi Tacos

PREP TIME:	COOKING TIME:	SERVINGS:
15 minutes	8 minutes	2

INGREDIENTS:

- 1/2 lb mahi mahi fillets
- 4 lettuce leaves
- 1 avocado, sliced
- Salsa

INSTRUCTIONS:

1. Season fish and cook in skillet until opaque, 4 minutes per side.
2. Serve in lettuce leaves with avocado, salsa.

Nutritional Facts (per taco):

- Calories: 150
- Fat: 7g
- Carbs: 4g
- Fiber: 2g
- Protein: 18g

Curried Mussels

PREP TIME:
10 minutes

COOKING TIME:
10 minutes

SERVINGS:
2

INGREDIENTS:

- 1 lb mussels
- 1/2 onion, diced
- 1 clove garlic, minced
- 1/2 can coconut milk
- 1 teaspoon red curry paste
- Cilantro

INSTRUCTIONS:

1. Sauté onion and garlic until softened.
2. Add mussels, curry paste and coconut milk. Steam until shells open.
3. Garnish with cilantro.

Nutritional Facts (per serving):

- Calories: 250
- Fat: 15g
- Carbs: 15g
- Fiber: 1g
- Protein: 18g

Crab Chowder

PREP TIME:	**COOKING TIME:**	**SERVINGS:**
15 minutes	20 minutes	2

INGREDIENTS:

- 4 oz lump crab meat
- 1 slice bacon
- 1/2 onion, diced
- 1 tsp curry powder
- 1/2 can coconut milk
- ½ Cauliflower

INSTRUCTIONS:

1. Sauté bacon and onion until browned.
2. Add cauliflower, coconut milk and curry powder. Simmer 15 minutes.
3. Puree until smooth, stir in crab. Heat through.

Nutritional Facts (per serving):

- Calories: 260
- Fat: 20g
- Carbs: 8g
- Fiber: 3g
- Protein: 14g

Chapter 9

COMPLIANT CONDIMENTS AND SAUCES

―――――――――

While the elimination phase of the Autoimmune Protocol excludes many common condiments due to allergenic ingredients, it is still possible to enjoy a variety of flavorful and nutrient-dense sauces, dips and dressings. Homemade condiments allow you to control ingredients to meet AIP guidelines. This chapter provides recipes for dairy-free mayonnaises, grain-free mustards, and nut-based pestos that can elevate simple meats and vegetables into satisfying meals. Immune-supporting herbs and spices are highlighted. Cultured vegetable pickles and kimchi also offer probiotic benefits. With just a few compliant ingredients and basic cooking techniques, you can create custom sauces to top or dip almost any food. The following recipes will help you enjoy restaurant-quality flavors while sticking to the strict AIP elimination diet.

Honey Mustard

PREP TIME:	COOKING TIME:	SERVINGS:
5 mins	None	2

INGREDIENTS:

- 1/2 cup Dijon mustard
- 1/4 cup honey
- 2 Tbsp apple cider vinegar
- 1 tsp dried oregano
- Pinch of unrefined salt (such as Himalayan Pink or Celtic Grey Salt)

INSTRUCTIONS:

1. Whisk all ingredients together in a bowl until smooth.
2. Store in a jar or container in the fridge for up to 1 week.

Nutritional Facts (per 2 Tbsp):

- Calories: 50
- Fat: 0g
- Carbs: 12g
- Fiber: 0g
- Protein: 0g

Creamy Dill Dressing

PREP TIME:	**COOKING TIME:**	**SERVINGS:**
5 mins	0 mins	2

INGREDIENTS:

- 1/3 cup full fat coconut milk
- 2 tbsp avocado oil
- 1 tbsp apple vider vinegar
- 2 tbsp dill, chopped
- Pinch of unrefined salt (such as Himalayan Pink or Celtic Grey Salt)

INSTRUCTIONS:

1. Mix all ingredients in a bowl.
2. Let it rest for 10-15 min.
3. Enjoy it.

Nutritional Facts (for a tbsp.)

- Calories: 54.5
- Fat: 5.9g
- Carbs: 0.6g
- Fiber: 0.2g
- Protein: 0.2g

Herbed Yogurt Cheese

PREP TIME:
8 hrs

COOKING TIME:
None

SERVINGS:
. 2

INGREDIENTS:

- 16 oz coconut yogurt
- 2 Tbsp olive oil
- 1 tsp dried dill
- Pinch of unrefined salt (such as Himalayan Pink or Celtic Grey Salt)

INSTRUCTIONS:

1. Line a sieve with cheesecloth and place over a bowl.
2. Pour in coconut yogurt and drain for 8 hrs in fridge.
3. Mix yogurt cheese with oil, dill and salt. Store in fridge.

Nutritional Facts (per 2 Tbsp):

- Calories: 30
- Fat: 2g
- Carbs: 1g
- Fiber: 0g
- Protein: 2g

Roasted Vegetable Dip

PREPARATION TIME:	**COOKING TIME:**	**YIELD:**	**SERVINGS:**
8 minutes	18 minutes	Approximately 3-4 cups	2

INGREDIENTS:

- 4 small or 2 medium-sized red root vegetables, peeled and diced
- 1 medium head of white cruciferous vegetable, chopped
- 1 teaspoon minced garlic
- Juice from half a fresh lemon
- 1/4 cup extra virgin olive oil
- Pinch of unrefined salt (such as Himalayan Pink or Celtic Grey Salt)

INSTRUCTIONS:

1. Preheat oven to 400°F (200°C).
2. Spread diced red root vegetables and chopped white cruciferous vegetable on separate baking sheets. Roast for 15-18 minutes or until tender.
3. Reserve about 1 cup of liquid from the roasted red root vegetables.
4. In a food processor, combine all ingredients with 1/4 cup of the reserved liquid. Process on high until smooth.
5. Adjust consistency by adding more reserved liquid as needed to achieve a smooth, dippable texture.
6. Allow the mixture to cool to room temperature before refrigerating.
7. Serve chilled with an assortment of fresh vegetable crudités such as carrot sticks, sliced radishes, and cucumber rounds.

Nutritional Information (per 1/4 cup serving, approximate):

- Calories: 70
- Protein: 2g
- Fat: 5g
- Carbohydrates: 6g
- Fiber: 2g
- Sugar: 3g
- Sodium: 150mg

Creamy Sauce

PREP TIME:	COOKING TIME:	SERVINGS:
10 mins	15 minutes	2

INGREDIENTS:

- 1 tbsp avocado oil
- 1 cup diced yellow onion
- 5 cloves garlic
- 1 cup coconut milk or cream
- 2 cups peeled and chopped white sweet potato
- ½ tsp apple cider vinegar
- ½ tsp truffle salt
- 1 tsp gelatin powder

INSTRUCTIONS:

1. Heat avocado oil in a medium pot over medium heat. Add onion and sauté for 4 minutes or until lightly browned.
2. Add garlic and sauté for 60 seconds until fragrant, being careful not to burn it.
3. Add coconut milk to the pot and bring to a boil. Add sweet potatoes and cook until tender, about 8 minutes.
4. Transfer the contents of the pot to a blender along with apple cider vinegar and truffle salt. Blend until pureed and smooth.
5. Stir in gelatin powder until well combined.

Nutritional Facts (per 2 Tbsp):

- Calories: 110
- Fat: 12g
- Carbs: 1g
- Fiber: 0g
- Protein: 0g

Ginger Carrot Pickle

PREP TIME:
30 mins

COOKING TIME:
None

SERVINGS:
16 oz (2 people)

INGREDIENTS:

- 8 oz carrots, sliced
- 1/2 cup white vinegar
- 1/2 cup water
- 2 Tbsp honey
- 1 Tbsp grated ginger
- 2 cloves garlic, minced

INSTRUCTIONS:

1. Combine all ingredients in a jar.
2. Refrigerate 30 mins to overnight before serving. Keeps for 2 wks.

Nutritional Facts (per 1/4 cup):

- Calories: 25
- Fat: 0g
- Carbs: 6g
- Fiber: 1g
- Protein: 0g

AIP Beet Ketchup

PREP TIME:	COOKING TIME:	SERVINGS:
20 mins	20 mins	2

INGREDIENTS:

- 1 tablespoon coconut oil
- ¼ large yellow onion, chopped
- 1 carrot, roughly chopped (about 1.5 cups)
- ¼ cup bone broth
- Pinch of unrefined salt (such as Himalayan Pink or Celtic Grey Salt)
- 2½ tablespoons beet juice
- 2 tablespoons water
- ¾ tablespoon honey
- ½ tablespoon apple cider vinegar
- 1 clove garlic
- 1 anchovy

INSTRUCTIONS:

1. Heat coconut oil in a small saucepan over medium heat. Once melted and hot, add onions and cook, stirring occasionally, until translucent, about 5 minutes.

2. Add chopped carrots, bone broth, and sea salt. Cook for 10-15 minutes, or until the carrots are tender. Remove from heat and let it cool slightly.

3. Transfer the mixture to a blender. Add beet juice, water, honey, apple cider vinegar, garlic cloves, and anchovy. Use a towel over the lid for safety and blend until smooth.

4. Pour the mixture into a container and refrigerate until chilled before serving.

Nutritional Facts (per 2 Tbsp):

- Calories: 15
- Fat: 0g
- Carbs: 4g
- Fiber: 1g
- Protein: 0g

Blender Hollandaise

PREP TIME:	**COOKING TIME:**	**SERVINGS:**
5 mins	None	2

INGREDIENTS:

- 4 ounces fresh basil (about 1 cup very tightly packed)
- 4 ounces fresh cilantro (about 1 cup very tightly packed)
- ½ cup extra virgin olive oil
- 1 lemon, juiced
- 1 clove garlic, peeled
- Pinch of unrefined salt (such as Himalayan Pink or Celtic Grey Salt)

INSTRUCTIONS:

1. Place all ingredients into a high-powered blender or food processor.
2. Blend on medium speed until the mixture reaches your desired consistency, using a tamper or stopping to scrape the sides of the processor as needed.
3. If the pesto is too thick, add additional olive oil gradually until desired consistency is achieved.

Nutritional Facts (per 2 Tbsp):

- Calories: 90
- Fat: 9g
- Carbs: 0g
- Fiber: 0g
- Protein: 1g

Apple Chutney

PREP TIME:	COOKING TIME:	SERVINGS:
30 mins	20 mins	2

INGREDIENTS:

- 2 apples, chopped
- 1 onion, chopped
- 1 cup cider vinegar
- 1/2 cup honey
- 1/2 tsp cinnamon

INSTRUCTIONS:

1. Simmer all ingredients in pot 20 mins until thickened.
2. Store in fridge up to 2 weeks. Enjoy with meats.

Nutritional Facts (per 1/4 cup):

- Calories: 70
- Fat: 0g
- Carbs: 18g
- Fiber: 1g
- Protein: 0g

Fermented Dill Pickles

PREP TIME:
10 mins

COOKING TIME:
None

SERVINGS:
16 oz (2 people)

INGREDIENTS:

- 1 lb pickling cucumbers
- 2 cloves garlic
- 1/2 cup water
- 1/4 cup vinegar
- Pinch of unrefined salt (such as Himalayan Pink or Celtic Grey Salt)
- Dill sprigs

INSTRUCTIONS:

1. Slice cucumbers 1/4 inch thick. Layer in jar with garlic.
2. Bring remaining ingredients to boil, pour over cukes.
3. Ferment 2-4 wks, refrigerate, enjoy within 2 months.

Nutritional Facts (per 1/4 cup):

- Calories: 5
- Fat: 0g
- Carbs: 1g
- Fiber: 0g
- Protein: 0g

Chapter 10

BONE BROTHS AND HEALING SOUPS

This chapter contains a selection of bone broth and soup recipes that are designed to support gut healing and provide comfort as part of an AIP lifestyle. The core bone broth recipes for chicken, beef and fish are easy to make and full of nutrients that can strengthen the intestinal wall and reduce inflammation. Going beyond basic broths, several satisfying soup options are also included like a Turkish egg drop soup, miso soup with shiitakes and bok choy for immune support, and a nurturing butternut squash soup. All recipes use only whole foods permitted on the Autoimmune Protocol and can fit conveniently into regular meal planning. The focus on simple preparations and ingredients highlights how healing nutrition in the form of bone broths and soups can be incorporated anytime throughout one's recovery journey.

Chicken Bone Broth

PREP TIME:

15 minutes

COOKING TIME:

12-24 hours

SERVINGS:

Makes 8 cups

INGREDIENTS:

- 3 lbs chicken bones
- 3 carrots, chopped
- 3 stalks celery, chopped
- 1 onion, chopped
- 3 cloves garlic, crushed
- 1 tbsp parsley
- 1 tsp black peppercorns

INSTRUCTIONS:

1. Place all ingredients in a slow cooker or stockpot and cover with water by 2 inches.
2. Simmer on low heat for 12-24 hours.
3. Strain broth through a fine mesh sieve and discard solids.
4. Chicken bone broth can be stored in the refrigerator for 3-4 days or frozen for 4-6 months.

Nutritional Facts per serving (1 cup):

- Calories: 20,
- Protein: 5g

Beef Bone Broth

PREP TIME:
15 minutes

COOKING TIME:
12-24 hours

SERVINGS:
Makes 8 cups

INGREDIENTS:

- 3 lbs beef or buffalo bones
- 3 carrots, chopped
- 3 stalks celery, chopped
- 1 onion, chopped
- 3 cloves garlic, crushed
- 1 tbsp parsley
- 1 tsp black peppercorns

INSTRUCTIONS:

1. Follow preparation instructions as for Chicken Bone Broth.
2. Strain broth and discard solids.
3. Beef bone broth can be stored and used similar to chicken.

Nutritional Facts per serving (1 cup):

- Calories: 30,
- Protein: 7g

Fish Bone Broth

PREP TIME:
15 minutes

COOKING TIME:
30-60 minutes

SERVINGS:
Makes 4 cups

INGREDIENTS:

- Bones and heads from 2-3 fish
- 1 carrot, chopped
- 1 stalk celery, chopped
- 1/2 onion, chopped
- 2 cloves garlic, crushed
- 1 tbsp parsley
- 1 tsp dill

INSTRUCTIONS:

1. In a saucepan, cover fish bones and vegetables with water.
2. Simmer for 30-60 minutes.
3. Strain broth and discard solids.

Nutritional Facts per serving (1 cup):

- Calories: 20,
- Protein: 5g

Miso Soup

PREP TIME:	**COOKING TIME:**	**SERVINGS:**
5 minutes	10 minutes	Makes 4 cups

INGREDIENTS:

- 4 cups bone broth
- 8 shiitake mushrooms, sliced
- 1 cup bok choy, chopped
- 2 tbsp white miso paste

INSTRUCTIONS:

1. In a saucepan, simmer mushrooms and bok choy in broth for 5 minutes.
2. Remove from heat and stir in miso paste until dissolved.

Nutritional Facts per serving (1 cup):

- Calories: 35,
- Protein: 3g

Thai Coconut Chicken Soup

PREP TIME:	**COOKING TIME:**	**SERVINGS:**
20 minutes	30 minutes	Makes 6 cups

INGREDIENTS:

- 4 cups bone broth
- 1 lb chicken breast, diced
- 2 carrots, diced
- 1/2 onion, diced
- 1 cup fresh cilantro
- 1 lime, juiced
- 1 (13.5 oz) can full fat coconut milk

INSTRUCTIONS:

1. In a pot, simmer broth with chicken and vegetables for 20 minutes.
2. Remove chicken and shred, then return to pot.
3. Stir in coconut milk and lime juice. Heat through but do not boil.

Nutritional Facts per serving (1 cup):

- Calories: 200,
- Protein: 18g

Italian Escarole Soup

PREP TIME:	**COOKING TIME:**	**SERVINGS:**
10 minutes	20 minutes	Makes 6 cups

INGREDIENTS:

- 4 cups bone broth
- 1 head escarole, chopped
- 3 cloves garlic, minced
- 1/4 tsp oregano

INSTRUCTIONS:

1. In a pot, sauté garlic in broth for 2 minutes.
2. Add escarole and seasonings. Simmer 15-20 minutes.

Nutritional Facts per serving (1 cup):

- Calories: 35,
- Protein: 3g

Turmeric Carrot Soup

PREP TIME:
15 minutes

COOKING TIME:
30 minutes

SERVINGS:
Makes 6 cups

INGREDIENTS:

- 4 cups bone broth
- 8 carrots, sliced
- 1 tsp turmeric
- 1/2 cup coconut milk
- 1 tbsp ginger, grated

INSTRUCTIONS:

1. Simmer carrots in broth until very soft, 20-30 minutes.
2. Purée with remaining ingredients until smooth.

Nutritional Facts per serving (1 cup):

- Calories: 50,
- Protein: 2g

Moroccan Lamb Soup

PREP TIME:
30 minutes

COOKING TIME:
2-3 hours

SERVINGS:
Makes 8 cups

INGREDIENTS:

- 6 cups bone broth
- 1 lb lamb shoulder, cut into 1" chunks
- 2 sweet potatoes, diced
- 1 tsp cinnamon

INSTRUCTIONS:

1. In a pot, braise lamb and potatoes in simmering broth with spices for 2-3 hours, until tender.
2. Remove lamb and shred, then return to pot.

Nutritional Facts per serving (1 cup):

- Calories: 150,
- Protein: 15g

Butternut Squash Soup

PREP TIME:	**COOKING TIME:**	**SERVINGS:**
15 minutes	30 minutes	Makes 6 cups

INGREDIENTS:

- 4 cups bone broth
- 1 butternut squash, peeled and diced
- 1 onion, diced
- 1/4 tsp sage
- Pinch nutmeg

INSTRUCTIONS:

1. In a pot, sauté onion in broth for 5 minutes.
2. Add squash and spices. Simmer until squash is tender.
3. Purée soup until smooth.

Nutritional Facts per serving (1 cup):

- Calories: 80,
- Protein: 2g

Tuscan Winter Vegetable Soup

PREP TIME:

15 minutes

COOKING TIME:

20 minutes

SERVINGS:

Makes 6 cups

INGREDIENTS:

- 4 cups bone broth
- 1 head cauliflower, chopped
- 4 cups kale, chopped
- 3 cloves garlic, minced

INSTRUCTIONS:

1. Simmer cauliflower in broth until tender, 15 minutes.
2. Add kale and seasonings, simmer 5 more minutes.

Nutritional Facts per serving (1 cup):

- Calories: 35,
- Protein: 3g

Chapter 11

FERMENTED FOOD FOR GUT HEALTH

This chapter focuses on fermented foods, which have long supported gut and immune health in traditional diets. We'll explore the gut benefits of home-fermented vegetables and dairy alternatives through their ability to influence the microbiome. Clinical studies show certain ferments can aid conditions involving gut inflammation.

Over 10 recipes provide nourishing fermented foods aligned with the Autoimmune Protocol. Enjoy traditional sauerkraut and kimchi along with lacto-fermented fruits. Innovative cauliflower, zucchini and beetroot ferments also adhere to strict AIP guidelines. Regular inclusion of these living foods can meaningfully support your healing through beneficial bacteria.

Homemade Sauerkraut

PREP TIME:	**FERMENTING TIME:**	**SERVINGS:**
15 minutes	2-4 weeks	Makes 1 quart

INGREDIENTS:

- 1 small head green or red cabbage, shredded
- 1 tbsp of unrefined salt (such as Himalayan Pink or Celtic Grey Salt)

INSTRUCTIONS:

1. Shred the cabbage into thin slices or chop finely. Place in a large bowl.
2. Sprinkle the salt over the cabbage and massage it in using your hands for 5 minutes until wilted.
3. Pack the salted cabbage into a 1 quart glass jar, pressing firmly to release its liquid. The cabbage should be submerged beneath the liquid.
4. Seal the jar and leave at room temperature (65-75°F) for 2-4 weeks to ferment. Check that the cabbage remains submerged by pressing a sealed bag inside the jar over the cabbage.
5. Refrigerate after fermentation is complete. Sauerkraut will keep refrigerated for months.

Nutritional Facts per 1/2 cup:

- Calories: 15,
- Sodium: 150mg,
- Potassium: 130mg,
- Vitamin C: 30% DV, Probiotics

Beet Kvass

PREP TIME:	FERMENTING TIME:	SERVINGS:
15 minutes	1-2 weeks	Makes 1 quart

INGREDIENTS:

- 1 lb beets, peeled and grated
- 1/2 lb carrots, grated
- 1 tbsp of unrefined salt (such as Himalayan Pink or Celtic Grey Salt)
- Water

INSTRUCTIONS:

1. Toss the grated beets and carrots with the salt in a large bowl.
2. Let sit for 30 minutes to draw out the liquid.
3. Pack the vegetables into a 1 quart glass jar, pressing firmly.
4. Fill the jar with filtered water to cover the vegetables, leaving 1-2 inches of headspace.
5. Seal the jar tightly and shake well to dissolve the salt.
6. Ferment at room temperature for 1-2 weeks. Check daily and press vegetables back under the brine as needed.
7. Refrigerate and enjoy within 1 month, adding water if needed to keep vegetables submerged.

Nutritional Facts per 1 cup:

- Calories: 30,
- Potassium: 450mg,
- Vitamin C: 15%
- DV, Probiotics

Garlic Dill Pickles

PREP TIME:
15 minutes

FERMENTING TIME:
2-3 weeks

SERVINGS:
Makes 1 quart

INGREDIENTS:

- 1 lb pickling cucumbers, sliced or whole
- 3 cloves garlic, halved
- 5 dill sprigs
- Brine:
- 4 cups water
- 3 tbsp of unrefined salt (such as Himalayan Pink or Celtic Grey Salt)

INSTRUCTIONS:

1. Wash and pack cucumbers into a 1 quart jar, adding garlic and dill.
2. Bring water and salt to a boil in a saucepan, stirring to dissolve salt.
3. Pour hot brine over cucumbers, leaving 1/2 inch headspace.
4. Seal jar tightly and ferment at room temperature for 2-3 weeks.
5. Transfer to refrigerator for up to 6 months. Enjoy!

Nutritional Facts per 1/2 cup:

- Calories: 5,
- Sodium: 210mg,
- Potassium: 85mg,
- Probiotics

Ginger Carrot Kimchi

PREP TIME:	**FERMENTING TIME:**	**SERVINGS:**
15 minutes	**1** week	Makes 1 quart

INGREDIENTS:

- 1 lb carrots, julienned
- 1/2 small onion, julienned
- 1 tbsp grated fresh ginger
- 2 cloves garlic, minced
- 1 tbsp unrefined salt (such as Himalayan Pink or Celtic Grey Salt)
- Water

INSTRUCTIONS:

1. In a large bowl, combine carrots, onion, ginger, garlic and salt.
2. Pack into a 1 quart jar and press firmly.
3. Fill jar with water, leaving 1/2 inch headspace. Seal tightly.
4. Ferment at room temperature for 1 week. Refrigerate to stop fermentation.

Nutritional Facts per 1/2 cup:

- Calories: 15,
- Vitamin C: 30% DV,
- Probiotics

Coconut Yogurt

PREP TIME:	FERMENTING TIME:	CHILLING TIME:	SERVINGS:
5 minutes	12-24 hours	6+ hours	Makes 2 cups

INGREDIENTS:

- 2 (400 ml) cans full-fat coconut milk
- 1/4 cup coconut yogurt starter culture

INSTRUCTIONS:

1. Warm coconut milk to 110°F in a saucepan.
2. Pour into a sterilized jar and add coconut yogurt culture. Stir to combine.
3. Ferment at 110°F for 12-24 hours until thickened.
4. Chill for 6+ hours before eating. Keeps up to 1 week chilled.

Nutritional Facts per 1/2 cup:

- Calories: 200,
- Fat: 20g,
- Probiotics

Kombucha Tea

PREP TIME:	**FERMENTING TIME:**	**SERVINGS:**
5 minutes	7-14 days	Makes 1 gallon

INGREDIENTS:

- 8 black tea bags
- 1 cup sugar
- 1 gallon water
- SCOBY and kombucha starter liquid

INSTRUCTIONS:

1. Brew tea with sugar and cool completely.
2. Add to container and top up with water.
3. Add SCOBY and starter liquid. Seal and ferment 7-14 days.
4. Enjoy or continue fermenting to desired flavor.

Nutritional Facts per 8oz:

- Calories: 35,
- Sugar: 8g,
- Probiotics

Tibicos

PREP TIME:	FERMENTING TIME:	SERVINGS:
5 mins	2-3 days	Makes 1 quart

INGREDIENTS:

- 1 quart coconut water
- 1/4 cup tibicos

INSTRUCTIONS:

1. Add tibicos to coconut water.
2. Ferment 2-3 days, taste testing daily.
3. Strain out and enjoy or refrigerate.

Nutritional Facts per 8oz:

- Calories: 50,
- Carbs: 12g,
- Probiotics

Rosemary-Peach

PREP TIME:
5 minutes

SERVINGS:
2 cups

INGREDIENTS:

- 4 cups peaches, diced
- 1 cup honey
- 1 sprig rosemary, stem removed
- ½ cup apple cider vinegar
- Sparkling water to serve

INSTRUCTIONS:

1. In a large mason jar, combine diced peaches, honey, and rosemary. Use a large spoon to muddle the mixture together. Cover the jar and refrigerate for two days, stirring occasionally.

2. After two days, blend the peach mixture until smooth. Strain the mixture back into the mason jar to remove any solids.

3. Stir in the apple cider vinegar, cover the jar, and refrigerate for another three days to allow flavors to meld.

4. To serve, fill a glass with ice. Pour enough of the peach mixture into the glass to fill it about ¼ of the way. Top off with sparkling water and stir gently before serving.

Nutritional Facts:

- Calories: 110,
- Carbs: 28g,
- Probiotics,
- Vitamin C 30% DV

Citrus-Basil Kombucha Ice

PREP TIME:	COOK TIME:	SERVINGS:
2 hours	2 hours	4 cups

INGREDIENTS:

- 2 cups fresh orange juice
- 2 cups fresh grapefruit juice
- ¼ cup basil, finely chopped
- ½ cup kombucha, any flavor

INSTRUCTIONS:

1. In a blender, combine orange juice, grapefruit juice, and chopped basil. Blend until smooth.
2. Pour the mixture into a 13x9" baking dish. Add kombucha and mix well.
3. Place the dish in the freezer for 30 minutes. After 30 minutes, use a fork to scrape apart any solid pieces that have formed.
4. Return the dish to the freezer and repeat the scraping process every 30 minutes for 2-3 more times, until the mixture has a crumbly, icy texture.

Nutritional Facts:

- Calories: 20,
- Carbs: 6g,
- Potassium: 70mg,
- Probiotics

Lime in Brine

PREP TIME:	**FERMENTING TIME:**	**SERVINGS:**
5 minutes	2-4 weeks	Makes 1 quart

INGREDIENTS:

- 8 limes, sliced
- 4 cups water
- 1/4 cup unrefined salt (such as Himalayan Pink or Celtic Grey Salt)

INSTRUCTIONS:

1. In a quart jar, dissolve salt in water.
2. Add lime slices and press to submerge.
3. Seal jar tightly and shake to mix.
4. Ferment 2-4 weeks at room temperature.
5. Refrigerate to stop fermentation.

Nutritional Facts per lime slice:

- Calories: 2,
- Potassium: 10mg,
- Probiotics

Chapter 12

DESSERTS AND SNACKS AIP RECIPES

━━━━━━━

While following the Autoimmune Protocol means limiting certain ingredients like sugars and grains, it doesn't have to mean depriving yourself of sweet treats. This chapter features 10 delicious dessert and snack recipes that are both nourishing and satisfying. From Coconut Yogurt Popsicles to Baked Plantain Chips, these AIP-friendly recipes prove that you don't need gluten, dairy or refined sugars to enjoy a snack or sweet indulgence. Best of all, since they incorporate whole foods like fruit, coconut and nuts, you can feel good about eating them without compromising your health goals. So whether you need an afternoon pick-me-up or a way to satisfy your sweet tooth, you'll find plenty of options here to enjoy without restriction.

Coconut Yogurt Popsicles

PREP TIME:

5 minutes

FREEZING TIME:

4 hours

SERVINGS:

6 popsicles

INGREDIENTS:

- 2 cups full-fat coconut yogurt
- 1/2 teaspoon vanilla extract
- 1/4 cup honey or maple syrup
- Pinch of unrefined salt (such as Himalayan Pink or Celtic Grey Salt)
- Fresh fruit such as berries, chopped Mango or banana (optional)

INSTRUCTIONS:

1. In a bowl, stir together the coconut yogurt, vanilla, honey/maple syrup and salt until well combined.
2. Fold in any fresh fruit, if using.
3. Pour mixture into popsicle molds and insert sticks.
4. Freeze for at least 4 hours until solid.
5. To serve, run molds under warm water for a few seconds to remove popsicles. Enjoy!

Nutritional Facts per popsicle:

- Calories: 50,
- Fat: 2.5g,
- Carbs: 6g,
- Protein: 1g,
- Fiber: 0g

Baked Plantain Chips

PREP TIME:	**BAKING TIME:**	**SERVINGS:**
15 minutes	20-30 minutes	. 2

INGREDIENTS:

- 1 very ripe plantain
- 1/4 tsp of unrefined salt (such as Himalayan Pink or Celtic Grey Salt)

INSTRUCTIONS:

1. Preheat oven to 325°F. Line a baking sheet with parchment paper.
2. Peel plantains and slice them lengthwise into 1/4 inch thick pieces.
3. In a small bowl, combine salt and chili powder.
4. Arrange plantain slices in a single layer on baking sheet. Sprinkle with seasoning mix.
5. Bake 20-30 minutes, flipping once, until crispy and edges are brown.

Nutritional Facts per 1/4 plantains:

- Calories: 70,
- Carbs: 17g,
- Fiber: 2g,
- Potassium: 350mg

Chocolate Avocado Mousse

PREP TIME:
15 minutes

SERVINGS:
2

INGREDIENTS:

- 1 ripe avocado
- 2 tablespoons carob
- 2 tablespoons maple syrup
- 1/2 tsp vanilla extract
- Pinch of unrefined salt (such as Himalayan Pink or Celtic Grey Salt)

INSTRUCTIONS:

1. In a food processor or with a hand mixer, blend together avocados, carob, maple syrup, vanilla and salt until smooth and creamy.
2. Refrigerate at least 1 hour before serving to thicken.

Nutritional Facts per 1/4 cup:

- Calories: 120,
- Fat: 8g,
- Carbs: 13g,
- Fiber: 5g,
- Potassium: 450mg

No-Bake Cookie Dough Bites

PREP TIME:

15 minutes

SERVINGS:

12 bites

INGREDIENTS:

- 1 cup coconut butter
- 1/2 cup honey or maple syrup
- 1 tsp vanilla
- 1/4 cup cacao nibs

INSTRUCTIONS:

1. Line a mini muffin tin with paper liners.
2. In a small bowl, mix together coconut butter, honey/maple and vanilla until well blended. Stir in cacao nibs.
3. Scoop dough into paper liners. Refrigerate at least 1 hour before serving.

Nutritional Facts per bite:

- Calories: 70,
- Fat: 4.5g,
- Carbs: 5g,
- Protein: 2g

Apple Crisp

PREP TIME:
15 minutes

COOKING TIME:
30 minutes

SERVINGS:
2

INGREDIENTS:

- 1 1/3 large apples, sliced
- 1 tablespoon + 1 teaspoon coconut butter
- 1 tablespoon + 1 teaspoon coconut flakes
- 2 tablespoons maple syrup

INSTRUCTIONS:

1. Preheat oven to 375°F. Place apples in an 8x8 baking dish.
2. In a small bowl, mix coconut butter, coconut flakes and maple syrup until crumbly. Sprinkle topping over apples.
3. Bake 30 minutes until apples are tender and topping is golden brown.

Nutrition Facts per serving:

- Calories: 110,
- Fat: 5g,
- Carbs: 16g,
- Fiber: 3g,
- Protein: 2g

Frozen Bananas

PREP TIME:	FREEZING TIME:	SERVINGS:
5 mins	4 hours	2

INGREDIENTS:

- 2 bananas, peeled and sliced

INSTRUCTIONS:

1. Place banana slices in a single layer on a baking sheet and freeze 4 hours or overnight until firm.
2. Transfer to a freezer bag and store in the freezer. Enjoy as a sweet treat!

Nutrition Facts per banana:

- Calories: 105,
- Carbs: 27g,
- Fiber: 3g,
- Sugars: 14g

Coconut Macaroons

PREP TIME:	**COOKING TIME:**	**SERVINGS:**
15 mins	20 mins	12 macarons

INGREDIENTS:

- 1 cup shredded coconut
- 1/3 cup maple syrup
- 1/4 tsp vanilla

INSTRUCTIONS:

1. Preheat oven 350°F and line a baking sheet with parchment.
2. Mix all ingredients together into dough. Scoop teaspoons onto baking sheet.
3. Bake 20 minutes until lightly golden. Cool before serving.

Nutrition Facts per macaroon:

- Calories: 35,
- Fat: 1.5g,
- Carbs: 5g,
- Fiber: 1g,
- Protein: 1g

Berry Shortcake Bites

PREP TIME:
15 mins

COOK TIME:
14 mints

SERVINGS:
6 bites

INGREDIENTS:

- 120 grams cassava flour
- 3 tablespoons coconut sugar
- ½ teaspoon baking soda
- ¼ teaspoon unrefined salt (such as Himalayan Pink or Celtic Grey Salt)
- ¼ cup palm shortening
- ½ cup coconut milk
- 1 tablespoon lemon juice
- ½ teaspoon vanilla

For the cream:

- 1 14-ounce can creamy coconut milk (preferably Arroy-D), refrigerated for at least 3 days
- 1 tablespoon maple syrup
- Fresh strawberries
- ½ teaspoon vanilla

INSTRUCTIONS:

1. Preheat the oven to 450 degrees F (230 degrees C) and line a baking sheet with parchment paper.

2. In a medium bowl, combine cassava flour, coconut sugar, baking soda, and sea salt. Stir to combine.

3. Add palm shortening to the flour mixture and cut in with a pastry cutter until pea-sized granules form. Do not overmix. Set aside.

4. In a small bowl, whisk together coconut milk, lemon juice, and vanilla. Add this mixture to the flour mixture and stir with a wooden spoon until just combined; the mixture will be slightly crumbly.

5. Transfer the dough to a lightly floured countertop or cutting board. Gently form into a large ball using your hands. Do not overwork the dough. Use a floured rolling pin to roll out to about 2 inches thick. Use a biscuit-cutter or the opening

of a small mason jar to cut out biscuits. Press down firmly without twisting the cutter. Transfer the biscuits to the prepared baking sheet, rework the dough gently, and continue until all dough is used (you should get about six 2-inch thick biscuits).

6. Bake for 14 minutes or until lightly browned. Remove from the oven and transfer to a wire rack to cool completely.

7. While the biscuits cool, prepare the cream. Scoop out the firm creamy top layer of the chilled coconut milk into a medium bowl (approximately half of the can for creamy brands like Arroy-D). Add vanilla and maple syrup. Use a handheld mixer to whip for about 5 minutes until the cream develops texture.

8. To serve, top each cooled shortcake biscuit with a dollop of cream and fresh strawberries.

Nutrition Facts:

- Calories: 200,
- Fat: 12g,
- Carbs: 22g,
- Fiber: 6g,
- Protein: 5g

Mango Pineapple Popsicles

PREP TIME:
5 mins

MAKE TIME:
5 hrs.

SERVINGS:
12 popsicles

INGREDIENTS:

- 16 oz chopped mangoes (about 2 cups)
- 16 oz chopped pineapples
- 1 cup water
- Juice of 1 lime
- 2 tablespoons honey, or more as desired
- ¼ teaspoon turmeric
- Optional: Additional fruit pieces for added flair

INSTRUCTIONS:

1. In a high-speed blender, pour water first for optimal blending.
2. Add chopped mangoes, pineapples, lime juice, honey, and turmeric to the blender.
3. Blend on high speed until smooth and creamy.
4. Pour the smoothie mixture into popsicle molds, leaving space at the top.
5. Freeze for about 1 hour, then insert popsicle sticks into each mold.
6. Continue freezing for at least 5 more hours or overnight until completely solid.
7. To serve, run warm water over the outside of the molds to release the popsicles easily. Enjoy these refreshing tropical treats!

Nutrition Facts: Per 1/2 cup:

- Calories: 180,
- Fat: 10g,
- Carbs: 18g,
- Fiber: 4g,
- Protein: 7g

Carrot Cake

PREP TIME:	COOKING TIME:	SERVINGS:
15 minutes	1 hour 10 minutes	8

INGREDIENTS:

For the cake:

- 150 grams cassava flour
- 100 grams coconut sugar
- 60 grams coconut flour
- 2 tablespoons arrowroot powder
- 1½ teaspoons baking soda
- ½ teaspoon cinnamon
- ½ teaspoon ground ginger
- ¼ teaspoon unrefined salt (such as Himalayan Pink or Celtic Grey Salt)
- Pinch of ground cloves
- ½ cup avocado oil
- ¼ cup maple syrup
- 2 tablespoons lemon juice
- 2 teaspoons vanilla extract
- 1 cup water
- 1 cup shredded carrots

For the frosting:

- ¼ cup melted coconut oil
- 2 tablespoons coconut yogurt
- 2 teaspoons maple syrup

INSTRUCTIONS:

1. Preheat the oven to 350 degrees F (175°C). Grease a 6-cup bundt pan with avocado oil and set aside.
2. In a large bowl, combine cassava flour, coconut sugar, coconut flour, arrowroot powder, baking soda, cinnamon, ginger, salt, and cloves. Mix well and set aside.
3. In a separate bowl, whisk together avocado oil, maple syrup, lemon juice, and vanilla extract.
4. Add the wet ingredients to the dry ingredients and stir until combined. Gradually add the water and mix until smooth. Fold in the shredded carrots.
5. Transfer the batter into the greased bundt pan.
6. Bake for 50 minutes, or until lightly browned. The cake will not rise much, which is normal for cassava flour baking.

7. Allow the cake to cool in the pan for 20 minutes. Carefully invert it onto a wire rack and let it cool for at least 40 minutes more.

8. In a bowl, combine melted coconut oil, coconut yogurt, and maple syrup. Whisk until smooth and thick but pourable.

9. Spoon the frosting over the cooled cake, allowing it to drip down the sides. Dust with cinnamon if desired.

10. Refrigerate the cake for 10 minutes to set the glaze. Serve chilled.

Nutritional Facts:

- Calories: 80
- Fat: 2.5g
- Carbs: 1g
- Fiber: 0g
- Protein: 10g

28 DAY MEAL PLAN

―――――

A balanced and nutritious diet is key to maintaining good health and well-being. This 28 day meal plan provides a variety of breakfast, lunch, dinner and snack recipes that are easy to prepare and suitable for most dietary preferences. The meals have been carefully selected to ensure proper nourishment with a good mix of proteins, whole grains, vegetables, fruits and healthy fats. Sticking to this meal plan will help keep you satiated and energized throughout the day while meeting your daily nutritional needs.

Day	Breakfast	Lunch	Dinner	Snack
1	Coconut Yogurt Parfait	Chicken Salad Lettuce Wraps	Slow Cooker Beef Stew	Baked Plantain Chips
2	Sweet Potato Toast	Rainbow Salad with Apple Cider Vinaigrette	Salmon Cakes with Remoulade Sauce	No-Bake Cookie Dough Bites
3	Bacon and Mushroom Frittata	Turmeric Soup	Herbed Lamb Chops	Apple Crisp
4	Salmon and Asparagus Scramble	Lox and Greens Salad	Shrimp and Grits	Frozen Bananas
5	Berry Chia Pudding	Mushroom and Kale Sauté	Bacon Wrapped Pork Tenderloin	Coconut Macaroons
6	Beef and Veggie Hash	Carrot Ginger Bisque	Tuna Poke Bowls	Berry Shortcake Bites
7	AIP Waffles	Lemon-Cilantro Roasted Brussels Sprouts	Grilled Chicken Wings with Homemade BBQ Sauce	Mango Pineapple Popsicles
8	Turkey Sausage and Squash Bake	Vegetable Bibimbap	Poached Whole Snapper	Carrot Cake
9	Tropical Smoothie	Butternut Squash Tacos	Baked Meatballs	Coconut Yogurt Popsicles
10	Leftover Meat and Veggie Fritters	Cauliflower Steaks	Italian Sausage Soup	Chocolate Avocado Mousse
11	Veggie Muffins	Kohlrabi with Shiitake	Cod en Papillote	Baked Plantain Chips
12	Lox and Greens Salad	Purple Potato Salad	Chili Lime Flank Steak	No-Bake Cookie Dough Bites
13	Ham and Pear Bowl	Creamy Coconut Greens	Scallop and Zucchini Skewers	Apple Crisp
14	Breakfast Casserole	Tropical Green Blast	Garlic Rosemary Rack of Lamb	Frozen Bananas

15	Coconut Yogurt Parfait	Rainbow Salad with Apple Cider Vinaigrette	Honey-Citrus Glazed Arctic Char	Coconut Macaroons
16	Sweet Potato Toast	Turmeric Soup	Protein Power Bowl	Berry Shortcake Bites
17	Bacon and Mushroom Frittata	Lox and Greens Salad	Shrimp and Mango Rice Bowl	Mango Pineapple Popsicles
18	Salmon and Asparagus Scramble	Mushroom and Kale Sauté	Ginger Chicken Meatballs	Carrot Cake
19	Berry Chia Pudding	Carrot Ginger Bisque	Baked Halibut with Herb Vinaigrette	Coconut Yogurt Popsicles
20	Beef and Veggie Hash	Lemon-Cilantro Roasted Brussels Sprouts	Citrus Chicken Kebabs	Chocolate Avocado Mousse
21	AIP Waffles	Vegetable Bibimbap	Caesar Salad with Roasted Salmon	Baked Plantain Chips
22	Turkey Sausage and Squash Bake	Butternut Squash Tacos	Turkey Cranberry Wrap	No-Bake Cookie Dough Bites
23	Tropical Smoothie	Cauliflower Steaks	Seared Tuna Salad	Apple Crisp
24	Leftover Meat and Veggie Fritters	Kohlrabi with Shiitake	Beef & Broccoli Stir Fry	Frozen Bananas
25	Veggie Muffins	Purple Potato Salad	Shellfish Boil	Coconut Macaroons
26	Lox and Greens Salad	Creamy Coconut Greens	Grilled Chicken Thighs	Berry Shortcake Bites
27	Ham and Pear Bowl	Tropical Green Blast	Mahi Mahi Tacos	Mango Pineapple Popsicles
28	Breakfast Casserole	Rainbow Salad with Apple Cider Vinaigrette	Curried Mussels	Carrot Cake

APPENDIX

SHOPPING LISTS

Proteins

- (Grass-fed) beef
- (Pasture-raised) chicken and turkey
- Wild-caught fish and fish (salmon, tuna, lox, shrimp, snapper, cod, scallop, arctic char, halibut, shellfish, mahi mahi fillets, mussels, crab)
- Bone broth
- Beef broth
- Chicken Broth
- Organic bone broth
- Fish Broth
- Bacon
- Ham
- Liver
- Lamb

Vegetables

- Leafy greens (spinach, kale, green salad, lettuce,)
- Non-starchy vegetables (broccoli, cauliflower, zucchini,)
- Root vegetables (sweet potatoes, beets, carrots, purple potatoes,)
- Mushroom
- Asparagus
- Sauberkraft

Fruits

- Berries (blueberries, raspberries, blackberries)
- Citrus fruits (oranges, lemons, limes)
- Avocados
- Pineapple
- Apples
- Bananas

- Pear
- Peach

Fats & Oils

- Extra virgin olive oil
- Avocado oil
- Coconut oil
- Coconut milk
- Ghee
- Avocado

Herbs & Spices

- Unrefined salt (such as Himalayan Pink or Celtic Grey Salt)
- Turmeric
- Ginger
- Cinnamon
- Garlic
- Onions

- Cilantro
- Rosemary
- Thyme
- Basil

Condiments & Sauces

- Apple cider vinegar
- Coconut aminos
- Dijon mustard
- Balsamic vinegar

Other

- Cassava flour
- Arrowroot powder
- Carob
- Maple syrup
- Honey
- Unsweetened coconut flakes
- Kombucha

SUBSTITUTION CHARTS FOR NON-AIP INGREDIENTS

Category	Traditional Applications	AIP Substitutions
Meats and Seafood	Meats and seafood are a staple for protein, omega-3 fats, and essential vitamins and minerals.	Use any kind of meat or seafood you aren't sensitive to. If sensitive to all seafood, increase intake of organ meats to compensate for missing omega-3 fats.
Nuts and Seeds	Nuts and seeds might appear in Paleo snacks (granola, trail mix), baking (almond flour, hazelnut flour), butters (sunflower seed butter, almond butter), seasonings (cumin, fennel seed), milks (almond milk), and oils (walnut oil, sesame oil).	Use coconut flakes in granola or trail mix, pumpkin or plantain flour instead of nut- or seed-based flours, coconut butter instead of nut butters, safe seasonings like ground ginger, turmeric, cinnamon, or sea salt instead of seed-based spices, coconut milk instead of almond milk, and avocado oil or extra virgin olive oil instead of nut- or seed-based oils. Use 1/4 the amount of coconut flour and add arrowroot or tapioca starch as needed.
Eggs	Eggs may appear in cooking (scrambled, poached) or in baking as binders.	Omit for cooking. For baking, use coconut oil or mashed banana (1/4 cup per egg), gelatin (1 tbsp mixed with 3 tbsp water per egg), applesauce, plantain puree, or pumpkin puree (1/3 cup per egg), or a combination.
Sweeteners	Sweeteners might appear in baking, beverages, and condiments.	Reduce the amount or omit entirely for a more AIP-friendly treat.

Peppers or Eggplant	Peppers are used whole (bell peppers, jalapenos) or as seasonings (cayenne, red pepper flakes).	Use zucchini and yellow squash instead of bell peppers or eggplant, and ground ginger instead of spicy peppers and pepper-based seasonings.
Potatoes	Potatoes are used as a side dish (mash, fries, baked).	Use cauliflower, parsnips, sweet potatoes, and beets to make mashes, fries, chips, or baked potato substitutes.
Tomatoes	Whole (in salads, soups) or in sauces and condiments (tomato sauce, ketchup).	Use cucumber, carrots, celery, or zucchini in place of tomatoes and no-tomato sauce instead of tomato sauce, paste, or puree.
Alcohol	In a drink, cooked in soups and sauces, and in extracts.	Omit in drinks. Use broth instead in soups and sauces. If present in vanilla extract, only use in recipes where it will be heated; otherwise, omit.
Condiments	Ketchup, mustard, mayonnaise, barbecue sauce, salad dressings, relishes, chutney, horseradish, and vinegars are often used as condiments.	Make your own condiments using AIP-friendly ingredients like no-tomato sauce.

MEASUREMENT UNIT CONVERSION TABLE

Category	Unit	Conversion
Volume	1 teaspoon (tsp)	5 milliliters (ml)
	1 tablespoon (tbsp)	3 teaspoons = 15 ml
	1 fluid ounce (fl oz)	2 tablespoons = 30 ml
	¼ cup	4 tablespoons = 60 ml
	1/3 cup	5 tablespoons + 1 teaspoon = 80 ml
	½ cup	8 tablespoons = 120 ml
	2/3 cup	10 tablespoons + 2 teaspoons = 160 ml
	¾ cup	12 tablespoons = 180 ml
	1 cup	16 tablespoons = 240 ml
Weight	1 ounce (oz)	28 grams (g)
	8 ounces	1/2 pound
	16 ounces	1 pound = 454 g
	2.2 pounds	1 kilogram (kg)
Length	1 inch (in)	2.54 centimeters (cm)
Temperature	Degrees Fahrenheit (°F)	(Degrees Celsius (°C) x 1.8) + 32
	Degrees Celsius (°C)	(Degrees Fahrenheit - 32) x 0.5555
Baking Pan Size	9x9 inch pan	23x23 cm
	8x8 inch pan	20x20 cm
	9x13 inch pan	23x33 cm
	Muffin tin	6 portions

RECIPE INDEX

REFERENCES

———

Alpert, J. S. (2005). The Inspector Calls: Causes and Effects of Inflammation. Boston, MA: Harvard Health Publications.

American Journal of Clinical Nutrition. (2023). [Study on natural sweeteners, blood sugar levels, and inflammation].

Amy, B. (2018). Mediterranean Diet Cookbook for Beginners. San Diego, CA: Bawa Publishing.

Azerrad, S. (2019). Understanding Autoimmune Diseases. Berkley, CA: Ostara Publishing.

Barrett, S. (2016). Vitamin D and the Epidemic of Deficiency. West Palm Beach, FL: Quill Driver Books.

Blaser, M. (2016). Missing Microbes. New York, NY: Henry Holt and Company.

Booth, S. L. et al. (2017). Vitamin K. Amsterdam: Elsevier Science Publishing.

Bruce, A. (2018). Healing the Leaky Gut. Seattle, WA: CreateSpace Independent Publishing Platform.

Chen, J. Y. (2020). The Autoimmune Wellness Handbook. New York, NY: HarperOne.

Chopra, D. & Tanzi, R. E. (2019). Super Brain. New York, NY: Harmony Books.

Davidson, J. (2017). The New Mediterranean Diet Cookbook. New York, NY: Avery.

Davis, W. (2015). Wheat Belly. New York, NY: Rodale Books.

Dengate, S. (2008). The Grain-Free, Sugar-Free, Dairy-Free Family Cookbook. Ridgefield, CT: Vashon Island Publishing.

Eat Dirt (2014). Why Microbes are Good for You. Berkeley, CA: North Atlantic Books.

Eisenstein, M. (2013). The Fermented Vegetables. Summertown, TN: Book Publishing Company.

European Journal of Clinical Nutrition. (2024). [Review on coconut products consumption and blood lipid profiles].

European Journal of Nutrition. (2024). [Study on unrefined salt use, mineral balance, and inflammatory markers].

Gregor, M. D. (2017). How Not to Die. New York, NY: Flatiron Books.

Holford, P. (2003). The Vitamin Cure. London, UK: Piatkus Books.

Journal of Clinical Investigation. (2023). [Study on fructose intake, insulin sensitivity, and inflammatory markers in autoimmune conditions].

Journal of Clinical Nutrition. (2023). [Study on tea consumption and inflammation in individuals with autoimmune conditions].

Journal of Lipid Research. (2024). [Meta-analysis on saturated fat intake, cardiovascular health, and inflammatory markers in autoimmune conditions].

Journal of Nutritional Biochemistry. (2024). [Study on omega-6 and omega-3 fatty acid intake and inflammatory markers in autoimmune conditions].

Koeth, R. A. et al. (2013). Intestinal Microbiota Metabolism of L-Carnitine, a Nutrient in Red Meat. Nature Medicine, 19(6).

Kresser, C. (2019). The Paleo Approach. Las Vegas, NV: Victory Belt Publishing.

Ludwig, D. S. (2018). Always Hungry. New York, NY: Houghton Mifflin Harcourt.

Mercola, J. (2011). The No-Grain Diet. Beverly, MA: Fair Winds Press.

Molecular Medicine (1998). Role of omega-3 fatty acids in neurological health. Greenwich, CT: JAI Press.

Nutrients. (2023). [Review on glycemic load, blood sugar levels, and gut health in autoimmune conditions].

Pendergrast, M. (2013). Uncommon Grounds. New York, NY: Basic Books.

Perlmutter, D. & Loberg, K. (2016). Grain Brain. New York, NY: Little, Brown and Company.

Perlmutter, D. (2015). Brain Maker. New York, NY: Little, Brown and Company.

Rangan, C. et al. (2019). Dietary Fats and Progression of Dementia. London: Academic Press.

Rouzaud-Sandi, M. (2020). Gut Health Cookbook. Avon, MA: Adams Media.

Tataranni, P. A. (2020). Why We Eat Too Much. New York, NY: Little, Brown and Company.

Vannice, G. & Rasmussen, H. (2014). Position of the Academy of Nutrition and Dietetics: Dietary Fatty Acids. Journal of the Academy of Nutrition and Dietetics. 114(1).

Vincent, S. J. (2018). The Mind-Gut Connection. New York, NY: HarperOne.

CLAIM YOUR BOOK BONUSES!

Thank you for purchasing our book. We hope you find it informative and enriching. To receive your exclusive bonuses, please follow the steps below:

1. Send an email to infolionsbooks@gmail.com.
2. In the subject line, please write: "Book Bonuses Request."
3. In the body of the email, include the title of the book you purchased.

Once we receive your email, we will promptly send you the bonuses associated with your book.

We appreciate your support and look forward to hearing from you!

Warm regards,

Lionsbooks

infolionsbooks@gmail.com

Made in the USA
Las Vegas, NV
21 October 2024

10139654R00116